OBSERVATIONS UPON THE NATURAL
HISTORY OF EPIDEMIC DIARRHOEA

OBSERVATIONS UPON THE NATURAL HISTORY OF EPIDEMIC DIARRHOEA

by

O. H. PETERS, M.D., D.P.H.

Cambridge

at the University Press

1911

CAMBRIDGE UNIVERSITY PRESS
Cambridge, New York, Melbourne, Madrid, Cape Town,
Singapore, São Paulo, Delhi, Tokyo, Mexico City

Cambridge University Press
The Edinburgh Building, Cambridge CB2 8RU, UK

Published in the United States of America by Cambridge University Press, New York

www.cambridge.org
Information on this title: www.cambridge.org/9781107634961

First published 1911
First paperback edition 2011

A catalogue record for this publication is available from the British Library

ISBN 978-1-107-63496-1 Paperback

PREFACE

THE causative agencies from which springs the plentiful harvest of child mortality in large cities may be conceived as a felted mass of rootlets almost inextricably intertwined. Those of poverty, bad housing, bad feeding, and neglect, may be severally recognized, but the extent of their interrelations with actual respiratory and alimentary disease—those to which the greater part of the mortality is referred—can be traced only with difficulty. It is the object of this work to aid in the labour of cutting away the matrix and entangling fibres and to lay bare the hidden ramifications of at least one important causative agency—epidemic diarrhoea.

This affection—if we accept provisionally the more novel and generally favoured conception as to its nature—is revealed as something very like an ordinary infectious disease, and one which permeates all classes, while the excessive mortality it gathers round itself in urban centres must be regarded as something superadded, owing to the vicious circle it forms with those baneful conditions of slum life mentioned above. On the other hand, its peculiarly intimate association with the circumstances of domestic life, from the continual faecal pollution of the interior of the household by infants and others, tends to make it more so than other affections of the kind peculiarly a class disease, and an especial scourge of dirty neighbourhoods. Dirty towns may however be saved from excessive mortality by a high percentage of breast-feeding.

A notable point in the interesting comparison that can be drawn between diarrhoea and typhoid fever is that, in accordance with their peculiarly opposite age-incidence curves, the marked and habitual depositing of infectious excreta within the household in the former disease may make the question of water-closet versus conservancy pan a matter of far less importance than in the latter.

This treatise, here reprinted from the *Journal of Hygiene* (Vol. X.), embodies both the practical observations made at Mansfield, and also the results of previous theoretical inquiry into the phenomena of the epidemic curve, representing three years of close research. Pressure of space required the abridgment of statistical matter in the first part and the exclusion of lengthy appendices dealing with every source of fallacy likely to arise in the collection of the data. These and all the original notebooks and analytical tables have however passed under the eye of the Editor, and it need only be said further that with the knowledge of the thoroughness and intensity of effort with which they were collected and of the constant guard maintained against all likely sources of error the writer is firmly convinced of the great value of the data as such, and that little seriously fallacious or casual has been admitted, either respecting the grouping of attacks or in other important particulars. The interpretation of the data, on the other hand, may of course at any future time be seriously called in question, and it was felt that an open mind should still be maintained with regard to the alternative theories as to the infectious or non-infectious nature of the disease. Nevertheless, if, from a severely practical standpoint, it be justifiable to eliminate all theoretical possibilities of which, at the present, we have no actual knowledge, there would certainly seem to remain a preponderance of evidence for the former—that is, for the conception of an infectious disease as outlined briefly above.   O. H. P.

LIVERPOOL, *March*, 1911.

CONTENTS

I. Introduction.

THE following observations upon the Natural History of Epidemic Diarrhoea were made in Mansfield during the summer and autumn of 1908. The fact that at the time the writer was engaged in preparing a paper—to which the present paper is to some extent complementary—upon the epidemiological relations of season and disease, lent special interest to the inquiries regularly made from the Health Department of the town into the circumstances attending fatal attacks of diarrhoea. Early in the season a more than usually extensive inquiry was made into one of these fatal attacks in an area where an outbreak of diarrhoea appeared to be spreading outwards from a group of old privy-middens. To test how far the condemnation of the latter was justifiable another area was taken on the other side of the town, where the houses were newly built and provided exclusively with water-closets; and records, collected by house-to-house visitation, were obtained of all cases of epidemic diarrhoea, whether non-fatal or otherwise, occurring in these localities. The inquiries thus begun were afterwards extended so as to embrace two fairly large districts, a chance of doing this being provided by the opportune postponement of the addition to the department of certain work of inspection which had been impending at the beginning of the summer. These districts were several times revisited and scattered observations were also made throughout the other parts of the town. During 1909, while there was no opportunity of making extended observations, there were valuable opportunities during the course of the routine inspections of the summer of testing and re-testing the principal results obtained during 1908.

The two areas thus systematically studied had a combined population of more than 2000, living in 413 houses. Of these houses 391 were each visited on several occasions during the season of 1908, from May to November, and 390 separate attacks of epidemic diarrhoea were recorded. Full details were obtained as to dates of attack, age incidence and age constitution of the population, milk-supply, sanitary arrangements, proximity to stables, and fly nuisance. Information as to meteorological and other relevant matters was also obtained.

The special value of this mass of raw material lies in the fact that it represents, not a record of scattered and unrelated cases, but a *complete and consecutive account of all diarrhoeal attacks* occurring in a large area and *throughout the course of the whole epidemic season.* A reference to the literature of the subject shows that substantial statistical records of diarrhoeal *sickness* are unfortunately still very scanty. They appear to be confined to those derived from the following sources: cases applying for medical relief at Poor Law establishments and hospitals: a few records of cases occurring in private medical practice: and scattered cases gathered by the Public Health staff from around the neighbourhood of fatal attacks. In three instances notification has been recently adopted. It would appear however from observations to be referred to later on, that only a small percentage of the total cases, with a disproportionate number of infants to adults, voluntarily seek medical relief, and by so doing afford an opportunity for notification to the Health Authorities; which suggests that in records gathered in that way allowance must still be made for a considerable margin of error.

The material was wholly collected by myself. The obscurity in which the clinical as well as the pathological entity of the disease is wrapped makes the gathering of such data a peculiarly difficult matter. And the trained discrimination necessary in deciding what to retain and what to reject makes it almost essential that, for purposes of research, the collection of such data should only be undertaken by a medical man. In the course of the subsequent analysis and preparation of the data for the following paper, it was seen from the outset that, though a little reconsideration of the original verdict might be perfectly legitimate in regard to many details collected, and greatly assist the force and clearness of argument, yet, owing to the difficulty of knowing where to stop such revision a rigid rule should be made, wherever doubt existed, to regard whatever conclusion was arrived at at the time of collection of the data as final.

General observations were also made in all parts of the town, including 13 other districts of a few score houses each evenly distributed throughout the Borough, and these will be referred to as support to conclusions drawn from the two large districts, the examination of the data from which will form the main body of this paper. Some confirmatory observations, as already stated, were made in the season of 1909.

Description and comparison of the two districts from which data were mainly obtained. The two districts, one triangular and the other quadrilateral in shape, can be compared in Charts I and II, App., where they are drawn to the same scale. They are situated on opposite sides of the town, almost due East and West from its centre, and the centre of one district is distant about a mile from the centre of the other. They exhibit as complete a contrast as could be obtained in the matter of site and sanitary circumstances, as the following brief résumé suggests:

The Triangular Area.	*The Quadrilateral Area.*
Houses : Many old houses (sandstone); also many newer ones (brick), from 8 to 12 years old.	*All new* houses (brick); none older than 4 years; much building still going on.
Rows of shops along the borders of the area.	Almost wholly residential.
Sanitary details: Many old privy-middens and pan (*pail*) *closets.* Greater part w.c.'s.	*All w.c.'s.*
Several stables.	Practically no stables.
Site : Well-manured Allotment Gardens formerly occupied site of newer houses.	Formerly *clean meadow* land.
Well-drained site (sandstone). Situated half-way up the slope leading from the centre of the town. Mean altitude 365 ft.	Well-drained site (sandstone and clay). Situated on the high ground surrounding the central part of the town. Mean altitude 420 ft.
Exposed to north and west winds only.	Exposed to all winds, particularly those from east.

Data as to the town of Mansfield.

Site : an upland situation, between the plains of the Trent and the plateaux of Derbyshire. It lies at the junction of the New Red Sandstone with the Magnesian Limestone.

Altitude : about 250 feet above ordnance datum in the basin-shaped depression at the centre of the town, rising in outlying parts of the borough sometimes to over 500 feet.

Industries : formerly cotton-doubling, hosiery, and agriculture. The collier population is now rapidly increasing.

Population has increased rapidly and is given as follows: 15,900 in 1891; 21,400 in 1901; 32,500 in the middle of 1908. The people of the town are a young, healthy stock, with a high *birth rate*, 33·6 in 1908; and a relatively low *death rate*, 13·8 in 1908.

Infantile Mortality Rate: 151 per 1000 births for the ten years 1898–1907, and 137 for 1908 ; against respective rates of 142 and 121 for England and Wales for the same periods.

Diarrhoea Mortality Rate: is not officially given, but, calculated from a total of 104 deaths in the last five years, 1904–8, it was 46 per 1000 deaths ; and 68 for 1908. The respective figures for the neighbouring city of Nottingham calculated from the death rate were 59 and 42.

Provision of Sanitary Conveniences, etc.: from data in the Health Report for 1908, the houses were in that year provided as follows :

> Midden-privies in   662 houses.
> Pan (pail) closets in   665   „
> w.c's in   5202   „

The midden-pits are generally provided with doors, and used as ashpits. The town is sewered throughout, and has a good water supply.

II. A Statistical Study of Age Incidence, Prevalence, Fatality, etc.

The statistical matter here presented is not of more than moderate proportions. However, the two large districts chosen originally for the contrast they presented in sanitary and other relevant matters, have been divided into sections, so that the returns for the various sections, and again the totals for each district, can be compared. Such comparisons have been included wherever space allowed. An appeal to internal evidence can thus be made. Again, it may be pointed out that the thorough disentangling and fairly complete weighing up of the numerous complex influences affecting the distribution of the disease, which have been effected throughout the paper, have provided the means of dealing very satisfactorily with quantities of data of quite microscopic proportions. Thus the writer would feel confidence in a demonstration of the main facts from material provided by the triangular district alone.

1. *Age Incidence.*

Incomplete returns from a number of houses have been excluded altogether. A number of possibly doubtful cases have also been omitted in preparing the "corrected table" (Table II *b*); but the difference thus produced is however practically negligible, and as it is not practicable to duplicate the various tables the data of the "uncorrected tables" have been used throughout the paper.

TABLE I. *Proportions affected of Parents* and Children in* Houses Attacked *with Epidemic Diarrhoea within the two districts.* "*Uncorrected Table.*"

	Fathers*	Mothers*	20 years & over	20—15	15—10	10—5	5—2	2—1	1—0	All persons
All persons	184	187	46	77	110	146	119	36	51	956
Persons attacked	67	67	11	9	20	40	61	30	33	338
Percentage incidence of diarrhoea.	36	35	23	11	18	27	51	83	64	35

TABLE II *a. Proportions affected of Parents* and Children in* All Houses *within the two districts.* "*Uncorrected Table.*"

	Fathers*	Mothers*	20 years & over	20—15	15—10	10—5	5—2	2—1	1—0	All persons
All persons	375	387	145	164	232	280	196	52	73	1905
Persons attacked	67	67	11	9	20	40	61	30	33	338
Percentage incidence of diarrhoea.	17	17	7	5	8	14	31	57	45	17

* Throughout the paper, "Fathers," "Mothers," and "Parents" include married persons both *with* children and *without* children, unless otherwise stated.

CHART A. *Age Incidence in Diarrhoea. The Sickness data is according to the above Tables I and II. The distribution at the various ages of every 100 Diarrhoea Deaths at Mansfield is also shown, calculated from the 138 deaths occurring during the five years 1904–8: it corresponds closely with that of London for the corresponding period.*

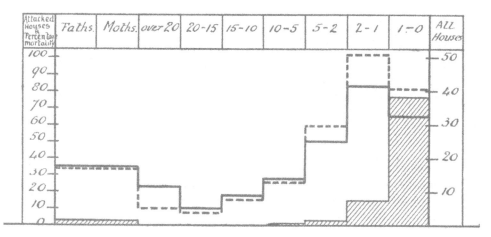

Percentage of diarrhoea Sickness in Attacked Houses only —— ; in All Houses ----- ; Mortality ▨ .

The most important points in the above chart and tables are the following :

(1) The result is somewhat at variance with the conception of the age incidence formerly held with regard to diarrhoea; and the attack age incidence is evidently quite different from the mortality age incidence.

(2) The totals under two years of age in the mortality table usually form about nine-tenths of the total number of diarrhoea deaths in the whole population, but in the observations here dealt with cases of sickness under two years form considerably less than one-fifth of all.

(3) Although the high attack rate amongst infants is the most striking feature of the age incidence, yet adults are not so very much less affected than young children: the proportionate incidence upon parents, children over five, and children under five, was roughly as 38 : 20 : 60 in attacked houses, and as 30 : 15 : 60 in all houses. The susceptibility of children decreases with increase in age to a minimum at the period 15—20 years; after which, even apart from the bringing up of a family and the resulting contact with susceptible children, there is perhaps a general increase up to extreme old age.

(4) Though the greatest fatality and the greatest attack incidence both fall upon children under two years of age, yet within that age period a great dissimilarity is found in regard to these matters: the mortality incidence is greater under 12 months than above that age, the incidence on the second year to that on the first being as 1 : 5 ; but the attack incidence in the second year is greater than that in the first year in the proportion as 5 : 4. As regards the comparative suscepti-bility of the youngest children, it is also worth noting that between

TABLE II *b*.   "*Corrected Table.*"   *Proportions affected with Epidemic Diarrhoea in* All Houses *within the two districts, separately and taken together.   Also, proportions of houses attacked.*

	Fathers	Mothers	20 years and over	20—15	15—10	10—5	5—2	2—1	1—0	All persons	Proportions of houses attacked
All persons	360	373	133	160	230	273	190	49	67	1835	391
Attacked persons ...	66	67	9	8	20	37	58	27	30	322	175
Percentage Incidence { Triangular area	19	18	5	5	6	9	30	65	46	16	45
Quadrilateral area	17	17	8	5	11	19	30	42	42	18	44
Both areas	18	17	6	5	8	13	30	55	44	17	44

two and three years of age the attack incidence has not yet fallen below that of the first year of life; the fatality has, however, decreased at this age to a very insignificant figure.

With regard to the results obtained by other observers, Ballard (1887–8) discusses the relative numbers of cases occurring under five years and over five years. At Islington he found it roughly as 6:1, and at Leicester 2·2:1. He inclines to the view that the former more truly represents the correct ratio, and gives his reasons for that belief (*ibid.* p. 26), which may be compared with the remarks on p. 151 of this paper. At Mansfield the ratio was as 2:1, almost the same as at Leicester, and from the manner in which the former data were collected, and from the above mentioned remarks, the writer regards this ratio as the more correct.

Owing to pressure of space the reasoned statistical inquiry as to age incidence has been abridged; only the conclusions arrived at, and the tables on which they are founded, being given.

(a) Variations in incidence at different ages.

The rise to a high incidence in older persons is to some extent affected by, but is probably not altogether determined by, their more frequent and closer association with susceptible infants (cf. Tables III (*a*) and (*b*), and V). There was some appearance of an abrupt rise in incidence at the age generally corresponding to the beginning of family life; but not a great deal of evidence as to a steady increase in susceptibility to diarrhoea sickness up to extreme old age, as suggested by the mortality data.

TABLE III *a.* *Some details as to the distribution of infection amongst Parents and Children in the two districts.*

Families collected into groups according as the eldest child was—	Parents affected, as a percentage of all parents	Parents affected in pairs, as a percentage of all parents attacked	Families where both parents remained unaffected, as a percentage of all families	Families where all the children remained unaffected, as a percentage of all families
Above 10 years	16·7	42	40	27
Under 10 years	17·7	50	51	12
Total	17	46	46	20
25 and upwards	7	50	50	50
25—20	15	} 41	41	27
20—15	21			
15—10	16	43	36	23
10—5	21	50	45	15
5—2	11	60	60	13
2—0	18	44	56	6

TABLE III *b*.

Amongst 145 " children " over 20 years, 11 persons, or 7 $\%$, were affected.
Amongst 17 uncles, aunts, and lodgers, 5 persons, or 17 $\%$, were affected.
Amongst 15 grandfathers and grandmothers, 5 persons, or 33 $\%$, were affected.

N.B.—Perhaps the latter, when they had not been attacked, were sometimes likely to have been forgotten, at the visit of inquiry.

The obviously high intrinsic susceptibility of young children is no doubt largely influenced, as regards which particular trimestral period is to present the maximum incidence, by the method of feeding (cf. p. 73).

At the age-period of lowest incidence, 15 to 20 years, there is still a moderate amount of intrinsic susceptibility. This is evidenced in many ways: e.g. 30 $\%$ of these cases were first cases, and a large number were the only cases occurring in their respective households (see also Table VIII).

Incidence on sex is approximately indicated in Table XI. There does not appear to be a great difference in incidence upon the two sexes (cf. Ballard, 1887–8, p. 29).

(b) *Statistical evidence for increased transmission of the disease amongst the members of a household owing to the close association of family life; demonstrating the occurrence of infection from a personal source.*

(1) The very high degree of *multiple infection occurring in households* is evidenced in Table IV.

TABLE IV. *Showing the amount and degree of multiple infection in all the 174 attacked households in the two districts. Alternate tabulations are presented below.*

Families containing—	Number of families	Percentage of all attacked families	Families containing—	Number of families	Percentage of all attacked families
1 case	91	51	1 or more cases	174	100
2 cases	44	25	2 ,,	83	47
3 ,,	23	13	3 ,,	39	22
4 ,,	8	4·5	4 ,,	16	9
5 ,,	4	2·2	5 ,,	8	4
6 ,,	0	0	6 ,,	4	2
7 ,,	3	1·7	7 ,,	4	2
8 ,,	1	·5	8 ,,	1	·5

(2) The marked influence of *association with susceptible children*, in increasing the incidence upon parents and other members of the family, is evidenced:

Firstly, in the results exhibited in Table V below:

TABLE V. *The* percentages attacked, *of* "parents" *and* children, *in all houses containing children*, according as to whether they do, or do not, contain infants (under 2).

	"Parents" in family groups, taken according as the age of the eldest child was—					All children above 2 years	Degree of dirtiness of attacked houses
	25—15	15—10	10—5	5—0	All parents		
In houses *with* infants (under 2).	23	20	23	14	19	17	55
In houses *without* infants (under 2).	18	15	17	12	16	16	52

Note the consistent nature of the greater affection of parents where babies are present, as displayed in the various family age-groups, questions of age susceptibility being eliminated: also the still more important fact that the higher incidence was more marked in parents than in other members of the family, owing unquestionably to the closer association of the former with young children.

As differences in dirtiness of households (cf. also Table XVIII) and in the number of children were not apparently sufficient to explain the facts noted, this table must be taken as a most important demonstration of personal transmissibility of diarrhoea infection.

The number of attacked children, per attacked house, other than infants, was much greater in houses not containing infants.

The inclusion of houses not containing children made no important difference.

Secondly, in the higher incidence upon parents in the "2—0 group" than in the "5—2 group," in Table III *a*. There was a greater number of affected infants in the first group.

Thirdly, in the abrupt rise in incidence noted, from unmarried persons over 20 years (Table II) to the youngest group of parents, whose average age was only about 26 years.

Fourthly, in Table III *a*, the tendency of both parents to be together affected increases at lower ages, as if on account of more frequent exposure to some common source of infection.

Fifthly, in the study—in the following section—of the frequency with which young children are responsible for the introduction of infection into a house.

Sixthly, in instances to be given later (cf. p. 101) of actual infection of parents from children.

(3) An examination of the effect of *the close association of married life* upon the mutual affectibility of parents, and of the influence of children upon one another, gave no definite results beyond reaffirming the already noted high degree of multiple infection occurring amongst the various members of the household.

(4) *The influence of parents upon children* calls for special mention, in view of the high incidence the former are subject to and of their habitual association with young infants in whom the deplorable mortality of the disease mostly occurs. Under the next heading it will be shown that in accordance with their high susceptibility, the parents play a considerable part in the introduction or first development of infection within the family.

(c) *Upon what members of the family rests the chief responsibility for the introduction of infection.*

(1) The *number* and *susceptibility* of the inmates of a house were found, as might have been expected, to determine, other things being equal, the degree of liability of that house to attack. Thus, houses containing the most susceptible units, children under two years, were found to have been proportionately more frequently affected than other houses (cf. Tables VI and VII).

Again, when the houses were arranged in successive groups according to the age of the youngest child, a gradually decreasing incidence was found in correspondence with the increased age and lessened susceptibility of the children (cf. Table VII).

The parents, the next most susceptible units after young children, are however necessarily excluded as a comparative factor, from their being common to most households; the influence exerted by the youngest part of the household thus practically alone holds the field as a differential factor, and most important contrasts are thereby afforded.

The greater the number of children in a family the greater is the liability of the household as a whole to attack (cf. Tables VII and XXI); and this result naturally follows, independently of the fact that houses with large families are also dirtier.

(2) An inquiry into *first cases*, i.e., as to the frequency with which any of the various units of the family was the first to introduce or to

TABLE VI. *Showing the proportionately greater incidence upon the houses containing infants (0—2) than upon the other houses.*

The first part of the Table indicates the proportions of attacked and unattacked houses amongst those containing and amongst those not containing infants, per 100 houses in each district and in the combined area.

Districts	Houses containing infants (0—2)		Houses *not* containing infants (2—0)		Total houses
	Attacked houses	Unattacked houses	Attacked houses	Unattacked houses	
Triangular	26	10	24	40	100
	36		64		
Quadrilateral	17	9	30	44	100
	26		74		
Both areas	21	9	27	43	100
	30		70		100

The second part of the Table indicates the proportions of attacked and unattacked houses per 100 houses containing infants, and per 100 houses not containing infants, in each district and in the combined area.

Districts	Houses containing infants (0—2)			Houses *not* containing infants (0—2)		
	Attacked houses	Unattacked houses	Total houses	Attacked houses	Unattacked houses	Total houses
Triangular	72	28	100	38	62	100
Quadrilateral	65	35	100	40	60	100
Both areas	69	31	100	39	61	100

Total number of houses containing infants (0—2)=119: all other houses=272. Cf. also the remarks as to the mass action of houses containing infants, p. 51.

TABLE VII. *Showing how the incidence upon houses varies according as they contain children of more or less susceptible ages. The incidence is also seen to vary according to the size of the family. The data as to dirtiness are included for purposes of correction. Cf. Table XXI.*

		All houses containing infants under 2	All houses containing children from 2 to 5 yrs., but none under 2	All houses containing children 5 yrs. or over, but none under 5	All houses containing children 10 yrs. or over, but none under 10	All houses containing children
Percentage of houses attacked		69	47	33	30	49
Percentage dirtiness of houses		57	55	44	41	52
Percentage attacked	Houses with 3 children & less	71	38	30	29	49
	Houses with 4 children & more	64	54	35	35	
Percentage dirtiness	Houses with 3 children & less	52	48	44	41	52
	Houses with 4 children & more	64	62	46	42	

TABLE VIII. *Showing what proportion, as a* percentage, *of all cases at each period were the* First Cases *in the season to occur within their respective households.*

Districts	Father	Mother	20 yrs. & over	20—15	15—10	10—5	5—2	2—1	1—0	All persons
Triangular	50	65	42	60	25	41	56	61	45	53
Quadrilateral	65	54	100	25	33	47	51	58	76	55
Both areas	58	58	63	44	30	45	54	60	57	54
Both areas (averages of 3 groups)	59			40			56			54

TABLE IX. *Showing that the tendency to figure as First Cases varies as the season advances, the tendency at some age-periods decreasing in intensity, and in others increasing. The distribution in the various age-groups is shown of 100 First Cases occurring in each half of the season. The data are from the two districts.*

	Fathers	Mothers	20 yrs. & over	20—15	15—10	10—5	5—2	2—1	1—0	Total first cases
First half of the season	24·3	22·5	6·3	1·8	3·6	6·3	17·1	11·7	6·3	100
Second ,, ,,	16·8	20·7	3·7	1·2	3·7	14·2	19·4	5·1	14·2	100
Percentage occurring in 1st half	56			38			47			50
Percentage occurring in 2nd half	44			62			53			50

TABLE X. *Showing the variation in incidence (expressed as percentages of all persons at the different age-periods) as the season advances. The data are from the two districts.*

	Fathers	Mothers	20 yrs. & over	20—15	15—10	10—5	5—2	2—1	1—0	All persons
First half of season	30	35	52	13	23	16	42	83	39	32
Second ,, ,,	33	31	28	8	10	33	56	76	71	33
First ,, ,,	33		52		18		50			32
Second ,, ,,	32		28		20		63			33
First ,, ,,	34			18			50			32
Second ,, ,,	31			20			63			33

develop infection, showed that this was generally in proportion to the degree of their susceptibility. Perhaps adults, it may be from their wider daily peregrinations, are a little more liable than others to become introducers of infection at the beginning of the season; and it is probable˙ that an important part is played by children in the second year of life, who were the "under ones" of the preceding diarrhoea season, in handing on the disease from that season, and lighting it up again in their respective households (cf. Tables VIII, IX and X). It is important to note also the greater tendency of certain age-groups to develop attack or to figure as first cases in the first than in the second half of the season. The early marked incidence upon ages 1—2 is in great contrast to the delayed attack of infants under one year (cf. Tables IX and X), the probable interpretation of which has just been given above.

TABLE XI. *Incidence on Sex. The sex-distribution of all persons attacked in the two districts. Not complete.*

Districts		Fathers	Mothers	20 years & over	20—15	15—10	10—5	5—2	2—1	1—0	All persons
Triangular	Males	32	—	2	2	1	9	17	6	8	77
	Females	—	32	2	2	5	8	13	11	11	84
Quadrilateral	Males	35	—	5	3	4	14	15	6	5	87
	Females	—	35	2	1	6	11	15	7	7	84
Both areas ("Uncorrected")	Males	67	—	7	5	5	23	32	12	13	164
	Females	—	67	4	3	11	19	28	18	18	168
Both areas ("Corrected")	Males	66	—	5	4	5	23	31	10	13	157
	Females	—	67	4	3	11	16	26	17	15	159
(Grouped)	Males	66			14		54		23		157
	Females	67			18		42		32		159

2. *Prevalence and Fatality.*

The very high incidence of diarrhoea throughout the districts examined was noted with some surprise. It was thought probable that for one district at least the conditions were such as to render it practically a diarrhoea-free district. The question might well be asked—Is the wholesale incidence of the disease here noted to be regarded as more or less usual in towns which are generally recognised as a little more than moderately affected with diarrhoea? Since comparisons between towns must at present be based wholly upon the death rate, it would be instructive to ascertain what ratio the total number of cases usually bears to the number of deaths, and whether that ratio is at all constant. It will appear that the proportion of non-fatal cases to fatal cases is probably much greater than that generally stated.

In the two districts, amongst the 338 cases or 407 separate attacks in the season, there were only two fatal cases. The distribution of these was as follows:

| | All cases | | |
	"Uncorrected"	"Corrected"	Fatal cases
Triangular area	166	156	2
Quadrilateral area	172	166	0
Combined area	338	322	2

Case Mortality   ·59 %

One other fatal case occurred in the western part of the triangular area, properly speaking however outside the area and amongst the houses, mostly shops, which were not visited.

It should be noted that even with this total of three deaths occurring within an area of the dimensions of the triangle, that district must be considered to have had rather more than its full share of deaths, since no area of similar size in the town had so many. On the other hand, the triangular and quadrilateral areas were no more severely affected with diarrhoea cases than many other parts of the town where observations were made. In the following season of 1909, certain parts of both districts which had a notable incidence in 1908 were again found to be almost as heavily affected, although 1909 was a cooler year with a very much smaller diarrhoea death rate. We are thus led to believe that there was nothing exceptional in what was found as to the great prevalence of cases, absolutely, and also relatively, to the deaths. Taking the lowest estimate, by dealing only with the corrected total for the one district— the triangle, in which all the deaths occurred, counting the three deaths and allowing a few cases for the unvisited areas around the margin, there would be at least 60 non-fatal cases to every fatal case. Taking the visited houses of both districts with the two deaths occurring therein, there were 161 cases to every death.

An average of about 100 cases to every death, whatever the results of future observations may be, would appear to be the only reasonable estimate to be deduced as regards the relation of sickness and mortality. If this be accepted and the mortality be multiplied by 100 to give the total cases of sickness, a rather high figure for the latter, that is, as regards our preconceptions of the disease, would be generally obtained.

The 34 deaths from epidemic diarrhoea and enteritis during 1908 at Mansfield would thus mean 3400 cases of diarrhoea in a population of 33,000, or that 10°/₀ of the whole population were attacked. In the neighbouring city of Nottingham, in a diarrhoeal year such as 1899, with 600 deaths, the 100 : 1 rule would mean 60,000 cases of diarrhoea in a population of 260,000, or 23°/₀ of all. This seems almost incredible, and it is probable that the ratio between sickness and fatality varies widely in different years and again in different towns. What statistics of sickness and mortality there are at present available suggest this; and the connection between mortality and sickness in diarrhoea is, moreover, a particularly loose one, a matter which will be specially referred to later on (cf. pp. 28 and 119). As regards Mansfield, however, during 1908, the writer saw no reason to regard 3400 cases, or 10°/₀ of the population attacked, as an over-statement of the prevalence of diarrhoea.

Inquiry into this question was made in a very thorough way, for besides the triangular and quadrilateral districts, there were 15 other localities, scattered over the whole town, where I made fairly extensive observations, to be referred to later on. In addition inquiries were made around the 34 fatal cases. Again, in visiting cases of the notifiable diseases which were unusually abundant in the autumn, or in calls made for other purposes, inquiries as to diarrhoea were also made, perhaps on more than 100 occasions. From this it will be understood, when the limited area of the town is considered, that I was able to obtain an intimate knowledge of the movement and dimensions of the epidemic in every part of the town, and that there were few streets even where I was not able to make more than a mere guess as to the precise degree of diarrhoea prevalence. The absence of mortality in the large quadrilateral area was by no means an exceptional case. In six other areas where I found diarrhoea to be very prevalent no deaths were recorded. Again, in several other areas foci were found where almost every house was attacked. The third area (Chart III, App.) is a sufficiently remarkable illustration of this. In short, there was every reason to believe that the suggested affection of 10°/₀ of the population did not by any means overshoot the mark. In the two large districts it must be remembered that as many as 18°/₀ and 17°/₀, respectively, of the population were affected. Judged by mortality, 1908 may be considered to have been a year of just fairly high prevalence. The average number of deaths for the five years ending 1908 was 27; and 1906 and 1908 had the greatest number, 34 deaths each.

3. *Variations in Age Incidence and Fatality with the Progress of the Season.*

(1) The variations in age incidence and in the tendency of different age-groups to figure as first cases, as the season advances, has already been referred to at the end of Section II, 1 (*c*) (cf. Tables IX and X, and Ballard, 1887–8, p. 40 *et seq.*).

(2) Ballard (1887–8, p. 20) found that the "ferocity" of an epidemic increased as the season advanced, as judged by the shortness of the time in which it kills its victim. At Mansfield the case-mortality appeared to increase towards the end of the season, thus agreeing with the somewhat late maximum affection of infants under 12 months (cf. Tables IX and X). The data with regard to this point are of course too meagre to base any conclusions upon, although since children under one were affected rather later than persons at other ages, the maximum mortality might also have been expected to fall later than the maximum prevalence of all cases. They may however be quoted as follows—the outbreak in the quadrilateral was apparently as late as most local outbreaks in the town :

	Prevalence in 4-weekly periods ending				
	July 4	Aug. 1	Aug. 29	Sept. 26	Oct. 24
Cases in Quadrilateral Area	12	47	73	42	19
Deaths in Town ...	1	1	8	11	9

III. Clinical Features, Immunity, etc.

1. *Special Clinical Features ; Diagnosis.*

The precise value of data as to attacks of diarrhoea, and of the conclusions drawn from them, will depend largely upon the degree of reliance that can be placed upon the *diagnosis* made at the time of their collection : and as regards the cases recorded in the above tables, some question naturally arises as to whether they were all undoubted attacks of epidemic diarrhoea. The characteristic features of epidemic diarrhoea, as regards the history of attack, are the occurrence of *diarrhoea, abdominal pain, vomiting, more or less well-marked depression, a tendency for the attack to extend for a longer period, and to take upon itself a more definite entity—so as to come to be regarded by the patient in the light of a real illness, than in the case of simple diarrhoea of a non-infective type.* As regards differentiation from the non-infective

2—2

type, in a large number of the latter there is simply looseness of the bowels without further accompaniment ; as in diarrhoea following slight digestive disorder, the administration of laxative substances, or over-indulgence in fruit.

The clinical picture of the specific affection is not however always complete, and several of the typical features may not be elicited. But a history of diarrhoea and just one other of the above-mentioned signs would, in certain circumstances, raise strong suspicion as to the infective nature of the attack. Of the latter signs, severe abdominal pain is one of the commonest in occurrence, and in consequence one of great diagnostic value, while of equal value in this respect is the characteristic and profound depression. Vomiting and prolongation of the attack are of course also important. As none, however, of the above signs are exactly pathognomonic of the complaint, we must, as in other infectious diseases, look to clinch the diagnosis, in a doubtful case, to the circumstances in which the case has occurred : that is, as regards the presence of the diarrhoeal season, and the occurrence of other cases in the same or neighbouring houses, especially if also closely related in point of time. It must be noted that the symptom of diarrhoea is not essential to the clinical picture : it is not constantly present.

Ten instances of the latter kind were incidentally noted, most of which had pain and vomiting or other symptoms : two cases have been abstracted from the data which the writer was disposed to include as instances of epidemic diarrhoea, in which severe abdominal pain was the only symptom. In the first instance, a father was doubled up with severe pain and felt sick, but did not vomit; five days afterwards his child, aged 3, developed a complete and typical attack. The second instance was that of a married couple without children; the wife had a severe attack of abdominal pain lasting two days, felt sick, and was constipated, but did not vomit; six days after the beginning of her attack the husband developed a complete and typical attack. In both of these instances there were at the time typical cases of the disease amongst the neighbours, and other suggestive circumstances. The two commonly mentioned symptoms, convulsions and change of colour in the stools, were of comparatively subordinate interest where four-fifths of the histories were not concerned with attacks in infants. There was of course every degree of mildness as well as of severity in the attacks.

As regards the existence of more than one specific disease, some of the evidence obtained appeared to suggest that this matter was worthy of consideration, but no definite conclusions were arrived at.

As the collection of data proceeded it became increasingly evident that it was not only desirable, but the only correct procedure, to throw the net rather widely than otherwise, and not to be misled by the light opinion of the attack held by the people themselves, or by the trivial causes to which they assigned it. *There could be little doubt but that practically the whole of the cases of the type collected were " epidemic," and probably also " infective " in character*, since they were practically non-existent at the beginning of the season, and decreased regularly as the temperature fell, while they were constantly related to other cases in the same or in an adjacent house. Experience taught that not too much notice was to be taken of "teething" and similar popular explanations, as evidence of a negative kind : a little careful inquiry would frequently reveal the presence of an undoubtedly specific attack of diarrhoea. Again, many cases of apparently simple diarrhoea in young children were found to suddenly develop in a very dangerous manner, so that the writer was forced to the conclusion that it was advisable not to regard lightly any history whatsoever of looseness of the bowels in infants during the diarrhoea season. Owing, however, to the great frequency with which digestive disturbances are known to occur in infancy, apart from specific diarrhoea, it might still be argued that little reliance should be placed upon the data relating to that period. To this it may be replied that either we must reject this conservative tendency to reduce the proportion of infective cases in infancy, or relinquish the other old conservative belief as to the much greater proportion of infants infected than adults ; for amongst adults the cases were always well marked enough to leave little doubt as to their right to be included amongst specific attacks. Further, the large amount of spread from infants to other members of the family must receive due consideration in this connection.

A discussion of *the popular conception* generally entertained *as to the nature and cause of the disease* is not only theoretically interesting, but is of some practical importance in view of the education of public opinion which must eventually be undertaken in this matter (cf. p. 157). As suggested above, the general tendency is to place it amongst the list of perfectly natural and trivial occurrences. Constipation on the one hand, and diarrhoea on the other, are regarded as disorders suitably adapted for home treatment, and not requiring special medical advice. The idea of infection is of course never entertained, and in laying about for a cause it is customary to seize upon the first suggestion that comes to hand. In infants it is invariably the teeth ; in adults, since it cannot be the teeth, it is fruit ; and of the different kinds of the latter, plums for preference. In the early summer, when plums are not available the cause is generally referred to strawberries. Among the causes assigned to demonstrably typical attacks of epidemic diarrhoea were medicine, currants, chocolates, fruit, teething, heat, and cold. It is true there seems to be a generally recognised obligation to name a cause for the attack, but having discharged that duty in the manner above indicated, and generally it appears with great mutual satisfaction to all concerned, patients and friends lapse into complete indifference upon the matter. Moreover, this not incorrectly sets forth the attitude of the general public, educated and uneducated alike, to what is in reality a very great scourge and a great sanitary reproach to the community at large.

It is necessary to insist upon certain matters of practical importance arising out of this popular indifference and complete unconsciousness to the actual existence of such a widespread and economically important disease as diarrhoea. The first relates to the great difficulty in obtaining histories of diarrhoea: the first enquiry is generally met by a negative reply, even only a few months after an attack; either the attack has already passed out of memory, or the fact is not grasped, that the insignificant occurrences recalled can possibly be the subject of inquiry. *An inexperienced enquirer, who unsuspectingly neglects constant, patient, and tactful cross-questioning, will certainly miss the greater part of the cases in the houses canvassed.* Nurses and medical men are themselves prone to pass over the specific nature of the complaint, and to regard as negative in a specific sense, histories such as, *e.g.*, that of being "subject to diarrhoea." The occasional negative observations as to spread in children's hospitals may possibly be found to be explained in this way (cf. note at foot of p. 106). Personally the writer would not rely upon his own recollections as to a previous negative history of epidemic diarrhoea.

It might be mentioned incidentally that in both adults and children there are a large number of attacks of great severity: so much so that it seems sometimes difficult to accept the suggestion that the attacks are on the whole more violent in warmer climates than with us. Many of the seizures in adults were of a severe choleraic type, with sudden onset, and intense prostration, accompanied by attacks of fainting, so that it sometimes seemed impossible that a fatal termination would be averted. In a large number of cases strong working-men were confined to bed for a fortnight or more; 12% of all cases, as stated before, sending for medical advice. No very complete figures as to confinement in bed were however collected.

Other features of the disease not so common as the above are—the passage of blood in some severe cases: a few of the attacks were of a markedly dysenteric type: jaundice was noticed in four cases, all in the quadrilateral district; two were related, as regards place and time, to each other and to typical diarrhoea attacks. Ballard (1887–8, pp. 15 and 18) mentions fugitive rashes, and refers to the diarrhoea occurring in some scarlet fever outbreaks: none of these rashes were met with; on one occasion however the spontaneous remark was elicited with regard to the diarrhoea prevalence, "What a lot of sore throat there is with it!"; moreover in six families, during the season, there was a history of sore throat associated in the same person with attacks of diarrhoea. In two of these cases bacterial swabs of the throat were examined, but none but ordinary throat organisms were found. The possibility of their being instances of "drain throat," or mild complicated cases of other throat affections, could not of course in so small a number be satisfactorily determined.

As regards the unsatisfactory and confusing titles conferred upon the disease: of the different combinations of the epithets "diarrhoea," "enteritis," "gastro-enteritis," "epidemic," "infective," and "zymotic," perhaps the most complete are the terms "zymotic gastro-enteritis," or "infective gastro-enteritis." But a title which purports to be a name, and nothing more, without reference to symptomatic or anatomical associations, as the name "cholera" has come to be regarded, would be, especially in the present state of our knowledge, by far the most satisfactory: and incidentally it must be confessed that, to one in daily close contact with the disease, the old title of diarrhoea, "English Cholera" or "Cholera Nostras," is the most satisfying one of all; for the clinical features of the disease are so peculiarly those of a "minor cholera."

2. *The Incubation Period.*

In a number of cases it was found possible to obtain facts as to the probable length of the incubation period, and this appeared to be frequently from 6 to 30 hours, although quite possibly it is sometimes longer. A history often obtained was that of exposure to infection on one day, followed by an attack on the day after; and less commonly, exposure to infection during the day with a sudden seizure during the same night. Bruce Low (1887–8, p. 127) describes four outbreaks of what closely resembled epidemic diarrhoea, and undoubtedly was so in one instance, in which the disease appeared to be directly communicated from person to person, and had an average incubation period of from 10 to 12 hours: in a number of cases, however, the attack developed on the day after exposure to infection. It might be supposed that, owing to the greater chance of exposure to such a risk, infection is most often contracted during the daytime; in which case, if the length of the incubation period happened to be about 12 hours, a larger number of attacks would occur by night than by day. This hypothesis was to some extent borne out by the facts: the probably correct time of onset was collected in 32 instances, and of these 18 began between 6 p.m. and 6 a.m., and 20 between 12 p.m. and 12 a.m. The incubation period appears from this to be nearer 18 than 12 hours in length, if exposure to the greatest risk of infection be supposed to occur between 6 a.m. and 6 p.m. Infection might of course have been contracted as long as an entire 24 hours, or several times that period, before this.

Another method of arriving at the solution of the matter is by noting that the reaction of deaths to temperature occupies from ten days to a fortnight. Since the average length of fatal attacks is sometimes nine days (cf. Table XIII), to which about two days must be added for registration, it follows that the incubation period of fatal attacks is generally less than three days.

3. *Duration of Attack: Acute and Chronic Cases.*

The duration of attack varies with age, and directly with the degree of susceptibility to attack, as indicated in Table II. Acute and chronic cases merge gradually into one another: there is apparently no clinical distinction to be made between them.

4. *Recurrence of Attack in the same Individual.*

(a) *During the same season.*

13 % of all cases had 2 or more attacks during 1908.
1 % „ „ „ „ 3 attacks „ „
1 case only had 4 attacks „ „

It was difficult to say whether many of these second attacks were not merely remissions of the first, owing to the smallness of the interval appearing to separate them. Such recurrent attacks merge imperceptibly into chronic attacks with remissions, which are very typical of chronic diarrhoea. Recurrent attacks also, generally speaking, vary with age, and are commonest amongst most susceptible persons.

TABLE XII. Duration of attack *of 100 cases at each age period.*

	1 week & under	1—2 wks.	2—3 wks.	3—4 wks.	Over 4 wks.	Total number of attacks	Average duration of illness in days	Number of attacks from which data are derived
Fathers	88	8	2	2	—	100	5·0	70
Mothers	86	9	3	1	1	100	5·2	75
25 & over	100	—	—	—	—	100	4·5	2
20—25	100	—	—	—	—	100	3·4	10
15—20	100	—	—	—	—	100	3·1	9
10—15	96	4	—	—	—	100	3·2	23
5—10	85	9	2	4	—	100	5·4	46
4—5	89	11	—	—	—	100	4·9	17
3—4	82	12	—	—	6	100	6·4	16
2—3	76	6	9	6	3	100	8·3	33
1—2	55	21	6	9	9	100	11·7	33
0—1	60	23	2	8	7	100	11·3	40
All ages (including Uncles, etc.)	82	10	3	3	2	100	6·3	394

TABLE XIII. Duration of attack, under two years of age, *compared, in* fatal *and* non-fatal *cases.*

	1 week & under	1—2 wks.	2—3 wks.	3—4 wks.	Over 4 wks.	Total	Average duration of illness in days
152 "deaths" (Blackburn)[1]	64	24	7	2	3	100	9·0
100 "deaths" of "children" (Manchester)[2] (93 were under 18 months).	50	25	8	5	12	100	?
73 "cases" (Mansfield) (non-fatal cases)	58	22	4	11	5	100	11·5

[1] Greenwood, *Blackburn Health Report for* 1906.
[2] Niven, *Manchester Health Report for* 1905.

TABLE XIV. *Cases at each age-period exhibiting* multiple attacks in the same season, *expressed as* percentages *of all cases at each age-period.*

								Under 5				
Fathers	Mothers	25 up.	25—15	15—10	10—5	5—2	2—0	5—3	3—2	2—1	1—0	All ages
7	13	—	11	10	12	16	15	9	24	20	12	13
	10									18		

(b) *In different Seasons.*

The recollection of previous diarrhoea attacks soon fades from the popular mind. Thus nearly half of previous attacks remembered occurred in the last four seasons. Of the total persons in two selected groups, *i.e.*, of (1) those who had a definite history of previous attack, and (2) those who were definitely stated to have had no attack; 59 % belonged to the first group.

5. *Immunity ; natural and acquired.*

The question of acquired immunity will be considered from evidence discussed in the paragraphs immediately preceding.

Recurrence of attack in the same season. On the one hand, it must be admitted that the percentage of cases displaying this feature is fairly high; on the other hand it might be urged that the greater part of the secondary attacks followed closely upon and were really not disconnected from the primary; and with regard to this fact it might be recalled that certain of those diseases conferring the highest degree of immunity have a very protracted and interrupted period of immunization. Thus typhoid fever with relapses may be said to consist of a series of separate attacks. In scarlet fever, a considerable percentage of cases develop a second attack within six to eight weeks of the onset of the first one. As regards diarrhoea, about 75 % of the second attacks followed within six weeks of the end of the first one, very possibly, in most cases, through the persistence and lighting up of the primary infection. Due importance must also be given to the fact that 86 % of cases appeared to be immune from a second attack; although, considering the plentiful distribution of diarrhoea cases in the two districts and particularly in certain foci, it might well be assumed that most attacked persons were exposed to infection on several subsequent occasions during the season.

Recurrence of attack in different seasons. There was a history of previous attack in about half. Considering therefore that in practically the greater number of cases the history of former attacks was probably forgotten, and recalling also the many facts already given as to the wholesale prevalence of the disease (Sect. II, 2), it might be safely concluded that in these mining and manufacturing towns of the Midlands most of the working-class population probably have several attacks of epidemic diarrhoea during their lifetime.

Duration of attack might also be supposed to have some relation to the question of immunity. And in perfect accordance with this it was found that both the duration of attack and the tendency to recurrence of attack in the same season varied directly with the degree of susceptibility to attack, all three thus being most marked in young children. The correspondence of the duration of attack in Table XII with the degree of susceptibility of different age-periods shown in Table II is remarkably exact, and incidentally is a striking testimony to the sufficiency of the data for a demonstration of the former point. The minimum in both cases is in the 15 to 20 years age-period. It might therefore be said that at this age-period the body shows greatest resistance, or the quickest reaction of immunization; expressed in popular everyday phraseology, it throws off the disease best at this age.

Fatality and severity of attack, there is no doubt, had also some relation to the question of immunity. Fatality of attack varies with the degree of susceptibility, being greatest in infancy and extreme old age; and immunity has already been connected up with susceptibility and duration of attack. Fatality in diarrhoea however does not depend only on the one factor, severity of attack, but also apparently very largely upon the physical resistance of the patient. Thus the effect of the greater severity of attack in infancy and possibly old age is magnified many times over by the low physical resistance at these age-periods. It cannot, however, be definitely stated that the severity of the symptoms apart from their mere duration was actually greater in infancy than, for example, in the 15 to 20 years age-period: there were of course no means of accurately testing this point. On the contrary, from the descriptions of the patients themselves, there seemed no reason to believe that at the latter age the attacks were much less severe during the few days through which they lasted; and the type generally met with was a short and rather sharp attack, frequently with violent diarrhoea, pain, and vomiting, and limited to about two or three days. The older patients, in accordance with their greater susceptibility, appeared to be perhaps more severely affected than the above, the attack being also sometimes considerably prolonged.

In summing up the above evidence as to immunity in diarrhoea, it must be remembered that, while the percentage of multiple attacks in the same or in different seasons was undoubtedly high, the chance of repetition of attack was much greater than that generally obtaining in any of the other infectious diseases, owing to the extraordinary and wholesale prevalence of the disease in question: a prevalence which, in the season, has no parallel with that witnessed in other infectious diseases, except in very extraordinary manifestations of the latter—where however the occurrence of second attacks, again, is usually common enough. That there is a moderate degree of immunity is evidenced not only by the large percentage of cases that, notwithstanding the above-noted ubiquity of infection, contrive to escape a second attack during the season; and by the suggestion in the epidemic curve of speedy collapse from exhaustion of susceptible material (cf. Sects. VII, 3 (*b*), II, 2 and 3); but also by the very great resistance offered to the disease by certain age-groups, particularly at 15 to 20 years and thereabouts, even in houses where infection is present. What is the precise nature of the great immunity evidenced at this age, whether natural or mostly acquired, it is difficult to decide. Finally, it is interesting to note that the variation of immunity with age in typhoid fever is exactly the opposite of that in diarrhoea, the ages of greatest and least susceptibility in the former being respectively the periods of least and greatest susceptibility in the latter.

6. *Some Clinical Aspects of the Mortality.*

Certain wide differences have already been pointed out between the *morbidity* age incidence and the *mortality* age incidence in diarrhoea, and the almost complete limitation of mortality to the first one or two years of life has been contrasted with the very general distribution of cases of sickness amongst all ages. But further than this, so large a part is played in this mortality by non-specific factors, such as actual pre-existing disease, or debility and bad nutrition related to defective social conditions, that the attack of diarrhoea almost comes to be regarded as rather an incident or accidental complication of the fatal illness, merely administering the finishing touch, like acute pneumonia in some other diseases. And thus the differences in diarrhoea, studied from the point of view of cases of sickness on the one hand, and of fatal cases on the other, are so great that they almost demand the separate recognition accorded to two different diseases. Relatively, one may say, in a free generalization, which must not be taken too literally— diarrhoea itself, *i.e.*, as regards morbidity, is a disease of health (cf. p. 148): but as regards mortality, it is a disease of ill health. Even a little over-statement of this matter, at the present time, should. be rather beneficial than otherwise; for it is only too apparent on following out the literature of the subject, how facts related almost exclusively to, and derived almost exclusively from, the mortality data, have over-coloured the true conception of the real disease. With the present rapid increase of sickness data, some readjustment of perspective must be looked for.

Two sets of observations, which afford a basis for the foregoing remarks and are well worth following out at length, must here be briefly mentioned.

Ballard (1887–8, p. 43 *et seq.*) found that in 332 fatal cases 57·5 % " had been either weakly from birth, or had been subsequently weakened by disease antecedently to their fatal diarrhoea attack." Niven, in the *Manchester Health Report* for 1904, pp. 179—181, found that in one lot of 111 diarrhoea deaths of children under 12 months, 75 had had " poor health " prior to the fatal attack, and 31 were said to have been in " good health," although the perfect soundness of all in the latter division is seriously doubted. The weakliness was due to the following causes : " failed to thrive " (14 cases); " previous illness " (12), tubercle being frequently suspected; " previous diarrhoea " (17), tubercle suspected in half of these ; colds and exanthemata (11); indigestion (11); 56 of these were probably insufficiently nourished. Only four of the 111 were being fed on the breast, the bulk of the others being fed on fresh milk and condensed milk. From the examination of another lot of 98 deaths (1905 Report, pp. 116—7) similar conclusions were also drawn. The results are summed up as follows : " It is very clear that the previous condition of the infant is one of the chief determining factors of fatal diarrhoea."

An examination of Mansfield mortality data also gave similar results. Perhaps one of the most important facts to bear in mind is that the change from mother's milk to cow's milk or other food, generally made between three and twelve months of age, is a physical feat on the part of the digestive organs only accomplished with difficulty ; and any disturbing cause, such as slight chronic or acute inflammation in the digestive tract, may be sufficient to render this at once impossible of safe accomplishment. Deserted by its digestive allies, the child readily succumbs to the strain of any exhausting disease, such as diarrhoea, which may supervene.

IV. SOCIAL RELATIONS.

The death rate from epidemic diarrhoea has been found by various observers to vary widely amongst different classes of the community, the better classes being relatively immune. It is not unlikely, although in view of the peculiar relationship of the mortality to sickness it does not necessarily follow, that the same rule holds good with respect to the general prevalence of non-fatal as well as fatal attacks of the disease. Should this be so, a comparative study of the different conditions obtaining in the various strata of society should give many useful hints as to the influences controlling the prevalence and spread of the disease. The following include perhaps the chief differences which might be supposed to distinguish the habits and conditions of life amongst the better classes in this connection: (1) greater general cleanliness: (2) a much smaller degree of closeness of personal contact: (3) greater care in the protection and preparation of food. It must be remembered that in the better class districts the common infectious diseases, generally, are recognised to be much less prevalent than amongst the artizan and labouring classes, presumably owing to the influence of the first two factors above mentioned. The first and third factors are dealt with in the two following sections in relation to diarrhoea. The second as to the effect of varying degrees of intimacy of personal intercourse will receive consideration in the present section.

The question as to the extent to which the *middle and upper classes* are subject to diarrhoea sickness is a very interesting one. No direct observations were made on this point, but from casual remarks gleaned the impression was received that the disease was not at all rare and perhaps more common amongst the middle classes than is generally believed, particularly when their houses are located amongst or have their rear premises bounded by small cottage property from which infection may pass to them. For many reasons, already discussed (p. 22), the presence of the disease amongst these classes does not come to the knowledge of the public; the cases being ignored or their details suppressed; the deaths also occurring perhaps comparatively infrequently. One can imagine, moreover, that diarrhoea might not have so secure a footing amongst the better class households, owing to the very solid opposition presented by the high degree of cleanliness there maintained; but that in years of special prevalence such areas might be subject to serious inroads of the disease from the humbler quarters of the town, in which it has been able to establish itself in the completely endemic form.

Socially, the population of both districts might be said to belong exclusively to one class—artizans, small tradespeople, and colliers. The wages were regarded as comparatively high, and likely to attract workmen of a high degree of physical fitness. The people were constitutionally of a strong and healthy stock, well-nourished, well-clothed, and prosperous; poverty being practically absent, and drink also as a cause of poverty; there being a tendency to excess rather in eating than in drinking. Thus the factors of drink, poverty, and insufficient food and clothing, which complicate the study of diarrhoea in the slums of large cities were absent, and the only difference of a social kind was as regards dirty and careless habits of living and in the care of food: but it should be noted that the differences amongst the various household units with respect to these factors were apparently as great as between each of the various social classes taken as a whole. Thus spotless cleanliness and an unexceptionable family ménage were frequently found side by side with gross filth and neglect. This shows how misleading general statistics as to prevalence in widely distant localities might be if collected without full knowledge of all the qualifying factors concerned. The quadrilateral area was notable as presenting, in passing from the S.E. to the N.W. corner, a gradual gradation from faultless household cleanliness and care in food, and comfortable living, to the other extreme. A general comparison of the two districts has been given in the introduction. That comparison will now be extended by the addition, as occasion offers, of further details in this and the following section.

1. *Houses, Rents, etc.*

The houses were of two stories, and mostly arranged in long terraces. The general interior arrangements, which were on a very uniform plan throughout the districts, were as follows (see Chart III, App.): There were three bedrooms upstairs and four rooms downstairs; the latter including a front sitting room, frequently not used, a kitchen generally used also as the eating and living room, a small scullery, and a small pantry, usually provided with fair means of lighting and ventilation. Bathrooms and additional bedrooms were found where the rents were above 6s. to 7s. From the kitchen and eating room a door led back into the scullery, and another, closely adjacent and to the side, opened immediately from the latter into the backyard. In the newer houses the rear part of the building was continued back behind the scullery, and was divided into two compartments to form the coal house and w.c., both communicating separately with the backyard. The rents were generally a good indication as to the condition and habits of the householders. They ranged from 4s. to 7s. in the triangle, and 5s. 6d. to 10s. in the quadrilateral. In the triangle more than three-quarters were between 5s. 3d. and 6s. 2d., with only six houses above the latter figure; in the quadrilateral nearly two-thirds were between 5s. 6d. and 6s. 3d., and three-quarters were between 6s. and 10s.; a third of the latter being above 8s. The higher rents in the latter district were not determined by the number and size of the rooms, but by the fact that the houses were newer, had larger gardens, were further from the centre of the town, and in a higher and more breezy situation. The nine houses in the triangle (Nos. 131—139) at 4s. to 5s. were very old

TABLE XV. *Showing the* House-Rents *per week, and the number of houses at the various weekly rentals in the two districts.*

Districts	4/-	4/3	5/3	5/6	6/-	6/2 & 3	7/-	7/6	8/-	8/- to 10/-
Triangular	9	4	10	64	84	5	5	1	—	—
Quadrilateral	—	—	—	53	12	68	24	—	14	38
Both areas	9	4	10	117	96	73	29	1	14	38

TABLE XVI. *Showing the weekly* House-Rents *in the various streets of the two districts.*

Triangular Area.

α Street—5/3.
β Street—5/6 to 6/2.
γ Street—East side 6/-; West side 5/6.
δ Street—5/6 to 6/-.

κ Street—Nos. 131—139, 4/-.
        Nos. 140—154, 5/- to 6/-.
μ Street—6/-.
        Nos. 155—158, 7/-.

Quadrilateral Area.

π Street—North side 5/6; South side 6/3 & 6/-.
ρ Street—North side 6/-; South side 79—86, 6/-; 87—93, 7/-; 94—107, 8/-.
τ Street—5/6.
σ Street—North side 7/-, Nos. 171—173, 8/-.
        South side 131—153, 5/6; 184—187, 6/-; 174—183, 188—213, 8/- to 10/-.

stone terraces containing sometimes only three rooms to the house, and though generally kept in a cleanly condition, were an inferior class of property. With the possible exception of the latter, however, there were no representatives in the two districts of the type of slum property found in large cities. Other details of the houses and of their situation are given in the Table on p. 6. They were mostly new; that is, built within the last ten years, and in accordance with recent by-laws. Generally speaking, the housing may be said to have been good, both as regards lighting, ventilation, and in most other important sanitary details. The differences in rent did not serve to mark very great differences in housing in the individual districts. As regards the majority of the houses, there was only the difference of a shilling in the rents of the different houses of each district. The houses over 8s. in the quadrilateral in σ Street were, comparatively, of a very superior class.

2. *Occupation.*

In both districts the people were mostly artizans or colliers receiving comparatively high wages. Factory hands and unskilled labourers were practically absent in the quadrilateral and were not numerous in the triangular area. The number of mothers employed away from home was quite negligible. As regards the possible influence of occupation upon the chances of infection, it was remarked in the section (II, 1 (*c*)) dealing with age incidence that sometimes the fathers appeared to bring infection home with them, perhaps from their work. Table XVII sets out, in the form of fractions, the numbers affected with diarrhoea over the total numbers employed at each trade. The figures are not complete for all houses in the triangle, nor for the southern half in the quadrilateral. They are, however, large enough to give some idea of the status and occupation of the people dealt with, and to yield an instructive comparison.

TABLE XVII. *Showing the* Occupation *of the* head of the family *in the various households of the two districts.*

The proportion of households attacked in each case is indicated by fractions, showing the number of houses attacked over the whole number of each occupation.

	Triangle	Quadril.	Total		Triangle	Quadril.	Total
Colliers	27/39	18/26	45/65	Agents	—	4/4	4/4
Grocer	3/4	1/1	4/5	Traveller	—	1/1	1/1
Baker	0/1	1/1	1/2	Contractor & builder	1/2	1/1	2/3
Butcher	—	0/1	0/1	Clerk	1/1	1/1	2/2
Storekeeper ...	0/1	0/1	1/2	Railway employees:			
Painter	1/1	1/2	2/3	Engine driver, fireman	—	5/11	5/11
Carpenter, joiner ...	1/2	1/1	2/3	Porter, guard ...	1/1	1/2	2/3
Fitter	—	2/2	2/2	Shunter, signalman	1/1	2/3	3/4
Foundry, moulding...	2/4	1/2	3/6	Police	—	1/1	1/1
Motor works ...	—	3/4	3/4	Mill: hosiery ...	2/5	3/6	5/11
Brickworks ...	3/3	1/2	4/5	Knitter	—	1/1	1/1
Tramcars... ...	—	1/1	1/1	Shoe factory ...	—	1/1	1/1
Corporation workman	3/4	—	3/4	Miscellaneous ...	3/10	1/2	4/12

Totals :—Colliers 45/65 ; *i.e.*, 69 % of such houses were affected with diarrhoea.

All others 57/92 ; *i.e.*, 61 % „ „ „ „

It would appear from this table that diarrhoea shows no limitation whatever to certain special trades and callings. In one instance, however, a special increased incidence might have been expected, viz., amongst colliers. Their special liability to typhoid has been several times noted, being due apparently to their careless habits of causing faecal pollution of the underground workings. The same might be expected to be even more marked in the case of diarrhoea, where such a practice is more a matter of sudden necessity than of carelessness. The households of colliers were affected in 69% of cases, against 61% in others; but against this may be placed the fact that colliers' houses were dirtier; and, particularly in the triangle, they included a higher proportion of houses containing susceptible infants (cf. Table XXII). A more satisfactory result is obtained by finding what proportion of fathers in the various occupations were affected. Amongst colliers 29% were attacked, and 19% in other callings. On the other hand, only 6% of colliers furnished first cases against 14% amongst all others, so that perhaps infection in uncleanly homes is most probably the real cause of the high incidence. At any rate the margin of cases is not sufficient, taking into account the incompleteness of the records, to indicate with any certainty that infection is brought home from the colliery much more frequently than from other places of employment. In other words, if much diarrhoea be brought home it is perhaps more probably due to the mere influence of personal association whilst at work, than to any special conditions in the work itself, apart at least from the method of disposal of the faeces.

3. *School Attendance.*

Bruce Low (1887–8) has described an outbreak of diarrhoea of an epidemic type arising from the use of a common privy at the village school. As regards personal contact, however, if the latter is of any importance at all the effect of school attendance should receive some consideration. In diarrhoea, it is to be noted, the reverse conditions hold to those met with in scarlet fever and diphtheria where school children embrace the most susceptible ages; for in the former disease, children of school age, particularly in the upper school, are at the time of life when most resistance is offered to infection. It is adults in their association at work who are the members of the family most likely to contract infection by contact with members of other households. Again, the incubation period of diarrhoea appears to be short and the onset sudden and unmistakable, and sufferers must perforce remain out of school, which is not nearly so often the case with diphtheria and scarlet fever. A good many records of school attendance were taken, but no indication was obtained as to special affection of any one school. In both districts four different schools were attended, the children often attending three or four different schools from the same family.

4. *Yards-in-common, and other factors determining closeness of human intercourse.*

Houses with backyards-in-common. There was a marked tendency for houses so related to be affected together, or to together escape infection. Yards common to several houses, from 2 to 15 in number, were found throughout the triangle. In the quadrilateral, yards-in-common were only found in the seven houses on the north side of π St.; in the last four houses on the south side of ρ St.; and in the 20 houses with backs adjacent, along the north side of σ St. These yards however provided little more than a narrow common entry from the street, owing to the railing off of garden plots at the back. A common entry, but of the kind providing very little opportunity of mixing of the neighbouring households, can also be made out on the charts in other parts of the same district. In this area, whatever the nature of the entry, the yards were always separately divided off; the dividing fence however was generally only three feet high with large interstices, of three or four inches, between the wooden palings; thus providing little hindrance to intimate association between the young children of neighbouring houses, as also between the parents. The practical relation of these facts to the question of diarrhoea incidence will be considered in a later section (Sect. VII, p. 89).

Structural arrangements of the back premises determining a specially close relationship between successive pairs of households.

Chart III shows the internal structural arrangements, already alluded to, typical of most of the terraced houses of the two areas. The effect of the backward prolongation of part of the rear premises deserves special consideration; the backward prolongation of two adjacent houses forming a deep recess or quadrangle, into the innermost angles of which the back entrance of each house opens. These doors, which lead directly into the scullery and kitchen, eating, or living room, thus open directly opposite each other and frequently at a distance of only 12 feet. The recess in the case of houses in the middle part of μ Street was only seven feet wide, and sixteen feet deep, with walls on three sides from 10 to 18 ft. high. An inner yard is thus formed, which must tend to restrict the movements of both the householders themselves, and possibly of fly-carriers, within this area; to the exclusion of their neighbours, who have to be reached by a considerable journey around the backward prolongation of the rear premises. It must also be noted that the doors of the w.c's open also opposite each other and into this area, the distance to the kitchen door of either house being also very little. The practical application of these facts will be considered in a subsequent section (Sect. VII, p. 91).

The data under Section IV may now be considered complete with the exception of facts as to personal intercourse between neighbours, and visiting between friends. Such data, if they could have been obtained, might have yielded important information, amongst other things, as to the occurrence of direct personal infection, and as to the transplantation of infection throughout a district.

V. SANITATION.

1. *Cleanliness of the household.*

The factor of household cleanliness has been frequently mentioned as probably holding an important place in the causation of diarrhoea, and it was therefore considered advisable and necessary to collect data under this heading. Marks were given, ranging from 1 to 5, to denote the degree of cleanliness or dirtiness of each home. The maximum of five indicated the greatest degree of dirtiness and untidiness, particularly as regards the leaving about of food exposed to the dirt and dust of the household. The minimum of one mark denoted that the family ménage was unexceptionable. The result of this enquiry showed that cleanliness of the home has an important relation to the comparative incidence of the disease in that it exerts a definite influence in warding off attack. It is important to record that as a means of gauging comparative dirtiness or cleanliness, the method adopted gave very reliable results (cf. p. 42). For the original data as to dirtiness Table XXVII *b*, App., should be referred to.

(*a*) The first method of presenting the data collected is as in Table XVIII which sets forth, amongst other things, *a comparison*

between the average dirtiness per house of those attacked and of those
unattacked with diarrhoea. The marks allotted to each house have been
added up and divided by the number of houses coming under each
heading. The averages thus obtained have been then expressed as a
kind of percentage, the maximum of five marks being equated to 100,
and the others to 80, 60, 40 and 20 respectively; the equivalent of
one mark being taken as 20, and not as 0, in order to facilitate the
handling of the data.

TABLE XVIII. *Showing the comparative dirtiness, expressed as a kind of
percentage (see text), in all households containing children, grouped according as to whether they do or do not contain infants (under 2 years), and
were or were not attacked with diarrhoea.*

The houses were divided into 5 classes; the dirtiest = 100; the cleanest = 20.
Cf. also Table VI.

Attacked and unattacked houses			All houses	Houses with and without infants (under 2)			
Both Areas:							
Houses attacked	With infants	55 } 54	52	57 {	55	Attacked	Houses with infants
	Without infants	52 }			62	Unattacked	
Houses unattacked	With infants	62 } 50		49 {	52	Attacked	Houses without infants
	Without infants	47 }			47	Unattacked	
Triangular Area:							
Houses attacked	With infants	58 } 58	58	60 {	58	Attacked	Houses with infants
	Without infants	57 }			65	Unattacked	
Houses unattacked	With infants	65 } 57		56 {	57	Attacked	Houses without infants
	Without infants	55 }			55	Unattacked	
Quadrilateral Area:							
Houses attacked	With infants	51 } 50	47	54 {	51	Attacked	Houses with infants
	Without infants	49 }			60	Unattacked	
Houses unattacked	With infants	60 } 44		44 {	49	Attacked	Houses without infants
	Without infants	41 }			41	Unattacked	

Tested in this way, the comparative excess of dirtiness in attacked
as against unattacked houses, expressed in the ratio 54 : 50, is not
great, but the result will be shown later to be qualified by various
factors; two important ones having relation to the presence of young
children and the size of the family. The qualifying influences of
association with dirty and highly attacked neighbours, and of the sharing
of "yards in common," also further tend to mask all distinctions between
the total dirtiness of attacked and unattacked houses.

It is sufficient however to note here the following points as regards
houses containing children.

Amongst all houses, the attacked were dirtier than the unattacked as 54 : 50.

Amongst all houses not containing infants (under 2), the attacked were again dirtier than the unattacked as 52 : 47.

Amongst all houses containing infants (under 2), however, the attacked houses were actually cleaner than the unattacked as 55 : 62 : although houses with infants were decidedly more dirty than other houses as 57 : 49, and these two facts were consistently observed in both districts. We might conclude, therefore, that houses containing infants were not more heavily attacked merely because they were dirtier than houses not containing infants; and that the influence upon diarrhoea incidence, dependent upon the presence of susceptible infants, is not on parallel lines with, and is powerful enough to subordinate to itself, that dependent upon dirtiness of the household. Attacked houses containing infants were, however, still dirtier than attacked houses not containing infants, in the ratio 55 : 52. The exceptional relations of the diarrhoea incidence to dirtiness in houses containing infants will be more fully discussed later on (Sect. V, 1 (*e*)), and, along with other things, the fact that breast-feeding saved a large number of infants living in the dirtiest houses of both districts from attack will be shown to satisfactorily dispose of the difficulty.

The importance of the above conclusions is emphasised by the fact that they are all borne out by the results obtained from the two districts taken separately as well as together. As regards houses without children, there was no difference in the degree of dirtiness of attacked and unattacked houses, the ratio being 37 : 37. But these houses were few in number, were scattered, and were practically all of one standard of cleanliness; 23 out of 28 were allotted either 1 or 2 marks, and only one was marked at more than 3. For this and other reasons it has been found convenient, and quite legitimate, to exclude them from most of the tables.

(*b*) A second and more striking method of presenting the data is shown in Table XIX, where *attacked and unattacked houses are compared as regards the relative numbers exhibiting the various degrees of dirtiness, as indicated by the index figure allotted to each house.* The result shows, as was to be expected, a preponderance of unattacked houses at the low indices, and a preponderance of attacked houses at the high indices; but an interesting feature is exhibited in the fact that by far the greater difference exists at the end of the table apportioned to the cleanest houses, the houses in the first column exhibiting a very special tendency to remain exempt (cf. p. 55). In comparing the relative numbers of houses attacked and unattacked under each index figure, a correction should of course be made as regards the relative percentages of attacked and unattacked houses in the district or

TABLE XIX *a*. *Showing the* number *of attacked and unattacked* households *containing children, exhibiting the various degrees of dirtiness, as denoted by the index figure at the head of each column.*

Districts	Numbers of houses which were	All houses containing children								Percentage of houses attacked & unattacked
		Indices of dirtiness					Indices of dirtiness			
		1	2	3	4	5	1 & 2	3	4 & 5	
Triangular Area	Attacked	5	20	25	11	6	25	25	17	53
	Unattacked	6	17	20	8	8	23	20	16	47
Quadrilateral Area	Attacked	11	26	20	9	2	37	20	11	45
	Unattacked	21	34	16	9	2	55	16	11	55
Both Areas	Attacked	16	46	45	20	8	62	45	28	48
	Unattacked	27	51	36	17	10	78	36	27	52

Districts	Numbers of houses which were	Houses *not* containing infants (under 2)				Houses containing infants (under 2)			
		Indices of dirtiness			Percentage of houses attacked & unattacked	Indices of dirtiness			Percentage of houses attacked & unattacked
		1 & 2	3	4 & 5		1 & 2	3	4 & 5	
Triangular Area	Attacked	10	15	6	40	15	10	11	73
	Unattacked	21	15	10	60	2	5	6	27
Quadrilateral Area	Attacked	23	14	6	39	14	6	5	62
	Unattacked	50	11	6	61	5	5	5	38
Both Areas	Attacked	33	29	12	40	29	16	16	68
	Unattacked	71	26	16	60	7	10	11	32

The percentage of attacked houses in these Tables refers only to those houses in which records of dirtiness were made.

TABLE XIX *b*. *Houses containing Infants (under 2), arranged into two groups according as the infant was fed on—*

Districts		Breast Milk		Cow's Milk	
		Indices of dirtiness		Indices of dirtiness	
		1 & 2	3, 4 & 5	1 & 2	3, 4 & 5
Triangular Area	Attacked	11	11	6	13
	Unattacked	3	*10*	0	2
Quadrilateral Area	Attacked	5	8	12	2
	Unattacked	1	*8*	4	2
Both Areas	Attacked	16	19	18	15
	Unattacked	4	*18*	4	4

districts considered : these percentages are given in the last column, the total number of attacked to unattacked houses in the two districts taken together being as 47 : 53.   Thus, before the numbers of attacked houses under the different indices can be compared with corresponding numbers of unattacked houses the former must be multiplied by $\frac{53}{47}$, or the latter by $\frac{47}{53}$.   The alteration however would be so slight that the correction need not be inserted, and on an inspection of the tables it is at once evident that it would not be sufficient to explain the differences noted.

Houses not containing infants were seen to show a still greater proportion of unattacked houses to attacked under indices 1 and 2; the contrast being greatly lessened when all houses were added together, especially in the triangle, on account of the directly opposite behaviour of houses containing infants, which have a much greater proportion of attacked than unattacked houses under 1 and 2.   Thus the irregularity noted in this class of house in Table XVIII again makes its appearance.

(*c*)   A third method adopted was to establish *a comparison between a group containing the cleanest and a group containing the dirtiest neighbourhoods* in the two districts.   More striking results were thus obtained (see Table XX), depending on the fact that clean and dirty houses were not evenly distributed throughout, but tended to be respectively grouped into a number of clean and dirty neighbourhoods. This was most marked in the long and drawn-out quadrilateral area, where the dirtiest houses were grouped towards one end of the district, and the cleanest towards the other.   The effect of this segregation of clean and dirty houses was to present a kind of *mass action* of cleanliness or dirtiness, apparently intensifying many times over the almost inappreciable effect of individual houses (cf. p. 54).   Thus where clean houses were distributed singly amongst dirty houses, differences in liability to diarrhoea were to a great extent masked or smothered; but where they were gathered together into a large group, they might be supposed to together present a solid phalanx towards the centre of which diarrhoea appeared to have greater and greater difficulty in penetrating.   Cf. π and σ Streets in the quadrilateral.

In Table XX*a* the two districts have been divided into a total of 33 sections : each section marking off a row or rows of houses in which there was a more or less constant tendency to one particular standard of dirtiness.   The cleanest and dirtiest sections have been then respectively grouped so as to, as nearly as possible, halve the total number of houses in each district.

The result shows that, even in the triangle, where the other methods failed to elicit any great contrasts, the excess of dirtiness and diarrhoea incidence in the dirty sections over that in the clean ones is very marked. Houses containing infants were, however, also more numerous in dirty sections: but it will be shown later that this only accounted in part for the greater diarrhoea incidence (cf. Sect. V, 1 (*g*)).

TABLE XX *a. Contrasting the* comparative dirtiness *and* comparative incidence *of diarrhoea of the* cleanest *and* dirtiest *groups of sections of the two districts.*

The two districts have been divided into 33 sections, and the cleanest 16 are compared with the dirtiest 17 sections. For comparison, the percentage of houses containing infants (0—2) is indicated. The table includes both houses with, and houses without, children.

	"Clean sections"			"Dirty sections"			Number of sections		Number of houses included in—	
	Percentage dirtiness	Percentage of houses attacked	Percentage of houses with infants (under 2)	Percentage dirtiness	Percentage of houses attacked	Percentage of houses with infants (under 2)	Clean	Dirty	Clean sections	Dirty sections
Districts										
Triangular	44	45	27	68	56	44	9	10	84	98
Quadrilateral	41	37	18	53	58	34	7	7	109	100
Both Areas	42	40	22	60	57	39	16	17	193	198

b. Showing the number of houses exhibiting the various degrees of dirtiness (as denoted by the dirt indices at the top of the columns) in Clean and Dirty Sections. Cf. Table XVI.

	All houses containing children		Houses *not* containing infants (under 2)		Houses containing infants (under 2)	
	1 & 2	3, 4 & 5	1 & 2	3, 4 & 5	1 & 2	3, 4 & 5
"Clean Sections"	37	20	18	14	19	6
	57	18	55	12	2	6
"Dirty Sections"	25	53	15	27	10	26
	21	45	16	30	5	15

(*d*) Before proceeding to draw conclusions from Tables XVIII, XIX, and XX, *the influence of the age-constitution, size, and occupation of the family upon the degree of dirtiness* must first be examined. Their special bearing upon the degree of diarrhoea incidence has already been studied in Sect. II and Tables VI, VII, XXI, and XVII, to which a reference might again be made.

From general observations it appeared that throughout the districts, with the almost complete absence of domestic help, household cleanliness constantly passed through certain definite evolutionary stages as the family grew up. The home of the young newly-married couple was generally very clean. In proportion as the number of children increased however, to some extent because of the inability of the mother to cope with the large increase of household work so entailed, the standard of cleanliness dropped lower and lower. With cessation of childbearing and entrance of the family into their teens an increasingly higher standard of cleanliness prevailed, probably owing to the operation of factors such as the following. The enforced activity of the mother during the years when the bulk of the family were young children, needing constant attention, has become a fixed habit, and as that burden has been gradually removed, her energies have been diverted into matters related more strictly to general cleanliness of the home. To this she is also impelled by the increasing self respect of the children as they grow up, particularly of the daughters, who are now also able to assist her; the wage-earning capacity of the family is also increased and they are able to provide many extra comforts and perhaps a more agreeably situated home. As the children leave home and the parents have only themselves to care for, the acquired habits of cleanliness remain, and the home is found to be, if anything, cleaner than at any other time. These facts are consistently borne out by the data of Tables XXI and VII, where the size, age-constitution, and dirtiness of the family are fully considered. Such complete conformity of the data with generally observed and accepted facts is at the same time important intrinsic evidence of its reliability; and it is largely for this reason that the latter have been outlined with such full detail.

The presence of babies in the household is one of the most important factors tending to dirtiness. This is not so marked with young parents where one or two babies comprise the whole family, but where childbearing has continued after the eldest child has reached 15 or 20 years it can generally be inferred that the family is too large to be kept at a high standard of cleanliness. As regards the size of the family, a point of some significance was that the number of children per family was much less in the quadrilateral area: 280 per 100 families with children, against 350 in the other district: the explanation certainly did not lie in the age or physique of the parents. The people of the quadrilateral district were more intelligent, and though of the same class, a somewhat superior type to the people in the triangle.

Their small families and their more disciplined habits contributed to make their district much cleaner than the other.

The above facts should be carefully followed out in Table XXI: it is there evident that the smaller families, containing three children or less, were consistently cleaner and less heavily attacked, except in the case of houses containing infants under two, which though still cleaner were more heavily attacked. Cf. also Table XXVII *a*.

There was also great variation in the degree of dirtiness of the household according to *occupation*. It was found in the preceding section under the heading of "occupation" (cf. Table XVII) that the houses of colliers were more often affected than those of persons following all other occupations taken as a whole. The chief reason for this, however, seemed to lie in the much greater dirtiness of houses of colliers; and, particularly in the triangle, in the greater proportion of their houses found to contain infants, as shown in Table XXII. Colliers' houses were mostly confined to a few neighbourhoods in each district; which, apparently from such houses providing the dirtiest dwellings

TABLE XXI. *Showing to what extent* dirtiness, *and* incidence of diarrhoea, *vary with* the size of the family.

Only houses containing children are included here, and only those in which data as to dirtiness were obtained. Cf. Table VII, and Table XXVII *a*.

		All houses containing		Houses *with* infants (0—2), and containing		Houses *without* infants (0—2), and containing		Houses with children all 5 years or over, and containing	
		3 children or less	4 children or more	3 children or less	4 children or more	3 children or less	4 children or more	3 children or less	4 children or more
Percentage attacked of all houses		47	51	72	62	36	45	34	35
		48		68		39		34	
Percentage dirtiness of	All houses ...	48	60	53	64	47	56	44	46
		52		57		49		45	
	Attacked houses	48	62	48	68	48	58	—	
		54		55		52			
	Unattacked ,,	48	54	65	59	42	52	—	
		50		62		47			

The two areas considered separately:

Percentage attacked of all houses	Triang.	53	52	83	66	38	38	38	36
	Quadri.	42	50	63	54	33	50	31	35
Percentage dirtiness of all houses	Triang.	52	66	55	65	51	67	—	—
	Quadri.	45	50	52	61	42	47	—	—

and from their more frequently containing susceptible infants, especially in the triangle, than other houses, proved to be localities showing the highest incidence of diarrhoea. Colliers' houses in the triangle were almost limited to a and γ Streets, on both sides of each street; and in the quadrilateral to π Street and the northern side of ρ Street.

TABLE XXII. *The relations between* occupation, dirtiness, *and* diarrhoea incidence.

Districts	Colliers			Other occupations			Numbers of houses from which data were collected	
	Percent. dirt.	Percent. of houses attacked	Percent. of houses containing infants	Percent. dirt.	Percent. of houses attacked	Percent. of houses containing infants	Colliers	Others
Triangular	72	69	60	44	57	31	39	40
Quadrilateral	55	69	30	43	65	28	26	52
Both Areas	65	69	47	44	61	29	65	92

(e) *The irregular relation to dirtiness of houses containing infants* (*under* 2) also requires special examination before final conclusions can be drawn from Tables XVIII, XIX, and XX. In these tables, amongst houses containing infants, the dirtiness of the unattacked houses was actually greater than that of the attacked; a result so pointedly the converse of that found amongst houses not containing infants, particularly in Table XIX, as to suggest that the element of chance enters to some extent into the question. The irregularity in the former class will now be critically examined.

In the first place, as appears from Tables XXI and VII, it so happened that the greater incidence of diarrhoea in houses containing infants fell upon the smallest, and on that account the cleanest, groups of families; whereas, in houses not containing infants, it fell upon the largest families, which also proved to be the dirtiest families. These facts were evident also in both districts, and most markedly in the triangle, especially in the clean sections of the latter. Moreover, in the same area, the highly attacked yards were, if anything, a little cleaner than the yards of low incidence, while they contained a much greater proportion of infants (cf. Table XXIV). Examining these houses individually upon the chart, it appears that 7 out of the 12 attacked houses with infants in the clean sections in the 1 and 2 columns, (Table XIX) proved to be in the comparatively clean μ Street, with an average family of 2·7 children, and an average dirtiness of only 37. In this case then, the irregularity was founded on an irregular distribution of infection, at least with regard to the degree of dirtiness. Another fact tending to produce irregularity is recorded in Table XXIII. The comparative percentage incidence of diarrhoea upon houses containing infants, in the " clean " and " dirty " sections, was as 69 : 69 ; being also about the same in both triangular and quadrilateral areas. On the other hand, upon houses *not* containing infants, there was a much smaller incidence in the clean sections, which after all might have been expected, being as 31 : 46 ; and similarly in the respective districts.

TABLE XXIII. *Showing percentage of houses attacked amongst—*

	Houses containing infants (under 2)		Houses not containing infants (under 2)	
	Clean sections	Dirty sections	Clean sections	Dirty sections
Triangular Area	73	71	29	42
Quadrilateral Area	65	67	33	50
Both Areas	69	69	31	46

This naturally tends to reverse the relations as to total dirtiness of attacked and unattacked houses in the two classes of households concerned ; and, should there be no differential influence from dirt, the total dirtiness of all attacked houses containing infants should be at least no greater than that of the unattacked. It would in fact be definitely a little less ; there being a fraction more of incidence upon clean sections. In the triangle therefore the irregularities in question may be largely attributed to the many irregularities observed in the relation of dirtiness to diarrhoea.

As regards the quadrilateral, however, the irregular relation amongst houses containing infants, of attacked and unattacked houses to dirtiness, which was observed in both clean and dirty sections, cannot be successfully disposed of along these lines. As a matter of fact, in the quadrilateral, the attacked houses of the above class, although cleaner, in the ratio 51 : 60, yet had somewhat larger families than the unattacked, in the ratio 2·9 : 2·4 ; where all such houses are included. It might here be added that the absence of records of dirtiness in some houses probably did not affect the issue.

We come now however to facts as to *infant feeding* which satisfactorily dispose of all doubts upon the matter. These apply particularly to the quadrilateral, where in dirty houses (indices 3, 4, and 5) breast-feeding was ten times more common, in proportion to feeding on cow's milk, than it was in clean houses (indices 1 and 2): the proportion of unattacked infants thus came to be much larger in dirty houses than in clean houses (cf. Sect. VI, 1). From Table XIX *b* it will be also seen that the excess of dirtiness of unattacked over attacked houses of this class could be satisfactorily attributed in each district to the large number of dirty houses (indices 3, 4, and 5) which were evidently saved from attack by the breast-feeding of infants; very little effect however being noted in clean houses.

It might be noticed here that the probable error for individual houses, in collecting the data, is large, the choice oscillating, *e.g.*, between 2 and 3, or between 3 and 4; *i.e.*, between 40 and 60, or 60 and 80. The practical inference from what has been said then is that houses containing infants tend to show, individually, some independence of dirt in developing infection; also, in the dirtiest sections, there is no greater proportionate incidence than in the cleanest, the percentages being as a matter of fact just equal (cf. Table XXIII). The greater total incidence upon clean houses is due to the irregular distribution of infection in clean sections, and of breast-feeding. Finally, it will be shown that within the attacked households of those containing babies, dirtiness still increased the incidence upon the other members (cf. Table XXVIII *b*). It may be concluded then that in the results as to houses *not* containing infants the element of chance played very little part, and that the opposite relation to dirtiness of houses containing infants may be ignored. Moreover, the number of the former class of houses was two and a half times as great as the latter, and therefore likely to yield more reliable results; and there was a constant and marked association of attacked houses of this class with greater dirtiness in all the analyses and tables presented, from Tables XVIII, XIX and XX, onwards.

(*f*) *The characteristic arrangement, in diarrhoea, of attacked houses in groups or clumps* (see Sect. VII, p. 88 *et seq.*), *the peculiar distribution of those clumps, and the qualifying influence thus brought to bear upon the effects of dirtiness*, is another matter that must be examined before proceeding further. The distribution of the clumps is frequently determined in a seemingly capricious manner, and apparently quite independently of the influence of dirtiness of houses containing infants, or of other recognisable factors. And these eccentricities of distribution of infective foci, it should again be noted, are regarded as peculiarly characteristic of the behaviour of an infectious disease. The intrinsic factors which determine the above distribution, primarily due to irregular distribution of infectious material or persons, will be discussed in another place (see pp. 95 and 137), but their qualifying influence upon the effects of dirtiness and of the presence of infants in each district may be studied in Table XXIV.

TABLE XXIV. *An analysis of* High Incidence *and* Low Incidence Sections; *as regards distribution of* attacks *and of* infants, *size of* family, *and degree of* dirtiness.

| | Percentage of houses attacked | Percentage of houses containing infants (under 2) | Degree of dirtiness | Size of family | Percent. of houses attacked in— | | Degree of dirtiness in— | | |
					Houses containing infants (under 2)	Houses not containing infants (under 2)	Attacked houses	Unattacked houses	Number of houses included
Triangular Area :									
High Incidence Yards	70	44	56	3·3	92	65	56	55	89
Evenly affected Yards	50	29	49	—	—	—	50	48	24
Low Incidence Yards	15	28	57	3·3	21	12	65	56	66
Quadrilateral Area :									
High Incidence Sections	78	26	49	2·8	96	72	49	47	104
Low Incidence Sections	16	24	43	2·1	34	10	49	42	105

TABLE XXV. *Showing the* increased incidence (*percent*) *of the disease upon all members of families situated within* High Incidence Sections, *compared with that found in* Low Incidence Sections. *The two areas are combined.* Attacked houses *only are included.*

	Fathers & Mothers	Children over 2	All persons
High Incidence Sections	33	28	35
Low Incidence Sections	26	21	28

N.B.—As many as 24 households are included in the Low Incidence Sections: their dirtiness was above the average of attacked houses.

To save needless multiplication of tables, a table showing the distribution of the attacked houses of the triangle within " yards-in-common " has been pressed into service here (cf. Table XXXII), since it so happens that the group of 20 high incidence yards includes practically all the clumps of attacked houses in the area, the low incidence yards representing the intervening rows of practically unattacked houses. Table XXIV, for the quadrilateral, has however been specially constructed for the present purpose, and allows a comparison to be made between the groups of high incidence sections—specially selected to embrace all the most highly attacked clumps of houses—and the groups of sections of lowest incidence.

From Table XXIV and others preceding, it is evident in both districts, firstly, that, although the distribution of diarrhoea was decided to some extent by the proportion of houses containing infants and to a less extent by dirtiness, the above-mentioned intrinsic factors, among which the influence of yards-in-common played a very important part in the triangle, were still more potent, and numerous irregularities in correspondence of the three factors above mentioned can be made out from a detailed study of the tables.

In the second place, it is shown that the differential effect of dirtiness was almost completely smothered inside the clumps; the dirtiness of attacked houses being no greater than that of unattacked. Outside the clumps, however, in the rows of low incidence, there was the usual greater incidence displayed upon dirty houses.

Thirdly, from Table XXV, it is evident that, within these high incidence clumps or sections, the incidence upon all members of the attacked families was much greater than upon members of households situated in low incidence sections.

In Table XXVI a few sections are collected in which irregularities in diarrhoea incidence, with regard to dirt, are very marked. The added details as to the presence of infants, as to the size of the

TABLE XXVI. Sections *of the districts presenting* marked exceptions to the general rule *that greater diarrhoea incidence is found in dirtier neighbourhoods, and less in cleaner neighbourhoods.*

| Districts | Dirty sections with *little* diarrhoea | | | | Clean sections with *much* diarrhoea | | | |
	Sections	Percentage dirtiness	Percentage of houses attacked	Percentage of houses containing infants (under 2)	Sections	Percentage dirtiness	Percentage of houses attacked	Percentage of houses containing infants (under 2)
Triangular Area	Houses 31— 35	72	0	0	Houses 155—162	33	50	12
	,, 136—139	90	25	50	,, 178—184	31	71	57
	,, 85—101	60	38	47	,, 11— 18	48	75	25
	,, 64— 66	70	0	33				
Quadrilateral Area	Houses 59— 78	57	30	50	Houses 87— 93	46	85	55
					,, 45— 58	44	64	28

Average size of family = 3·7 children   Average size of family = 2·6 children families and their possible lack of immunity, and as to the sharing of common yards, show that none of these factors were sufficient to explain those occurrences.

The much smaller difference in dirtiness of attacked and unattacked houses in the triangle than in the quadrilateral, noted above, probably largely depends upon the different arrangement of the houses in the two areas. Thus, while in the quadrilateral the rows of houses line parallel streets and are further apart and the district is larger and more drawn out, in the triangle the district is, so to speak, folded round upon itself into as compact a mass of streets and houses as possible, the major part of the houses being much more closely placed than in the other district. Thus dirty and clean rows of houses, which are found sprinkled in alternate groups over the whole district, are brought into very close contact, with consequent easier passage of infection from one to the other, while the distinctions due to differences in cleanliness are to a great extent lost; in contrast to the arrangement in the quadrilateral, where the segregation of clean and dirty rows towards different ends of the district, out of reach of one another's qualifying influence, is so well fitted to present the greatest contrasts of the kind under notice. Again, in the triangle the capricious distribution of infection, largely influenced by the presence of yards-in-common, has occurred to a very marked degree (cf. the examples in Table XXVI), and several negative results, as regards the influence of dirt, size of family, etc., are to be wholly attributed to this fact (cf. Table XXVII).

(*g*) *The amount of correlation between the respective proportions of diarrhoea, of infants, and of dirtiness, throughout the various parts of the districts.* The difficult problem of the disentangling of the respective influences upon diarrhoea prevalence, of dirtiness and of houses containing infants, may be satisfactorily accomplished by working out the amount of correlation between the three separate factors from the data of the individual houses (cf. Table XXVII *b*, App.)—correlating the positive or negative history of attack of each house with its index figure of dirt, and also with the number of infants (under 2) it contains. Again, the correlation of diarrhoea and dirtiness with a fourth quantity—the size of the family, was obtained; in this case the number of children per house was used, the two parents being practically constant for all houses[1].

---

[1] I am indebted for some valuable criticisms and suggestions upon these matters to the kindness of Mr David Heron, Galton Eugenics Laboratory, London, and Dr Cameron Gibson, Municipal Offices, Liverpool.

TABLE XXVII *a*. *The Coefficients of Correlation amongst the individual houses of the districts, between two sets of factors, including for each house* (1) *the positive or negative history of attack,* (2) *the number of infants* (under 2), (3) *the individual index figure of dirtiness, and* (4) *the size of the family* (number of children). *Cf. also Table XXI.*

	Infants and dirtiness	Infants and diarrhoea	Diarrhoea and dirtiness	Diarrhoea and dirtiness (pure)
Triangular Area	0·22	0·31	0·02	− 0·04
Quadrilateral Area	0·21	0·22	0·13	0·09
Both Areas	0·215	0·276	0·083	0·025

	Size of family and dirtiness	Size of family and diarrhoea	Diarrhoea and dirtiness	Diarrhoea and dirtiness (pure)
Triangular Area	0·35	− 0·01	0·02	0·02
Quadrilateral Area	0·20	0·17	0·13	0·10
Both Areas	0·307	0·062	0·083	0·067

Houses not containing infants (under 2):

	Size of family and dirtiness	Size of family and diarrhoea	Diarrhoea and dirtiness	Diarrhoea and dirtiness (pure)
Triangular Area	0·37	− 0·09	0·01	0·05
Quadrilateral Area	0·16	0·18	0·17	0·14
Both Areas	0·287	0·057	0·088	0·078

Table XXVII *a* presents the two sets of coefficients of correlation thus obtained: in the fourth column is shown the pure correlation between dirt and diarrhoea, *i.e.,* after the correlation values which depend wholly upon the mutual correlations of infants and diarrhoea in the first set, and of size of family and diarrhoea in the second set, have been eliminated. The results are instructive, although in the so-called pure correlation value in each set the influence of the fourth factor, and probably of other unestimated factors as well, has not been eliminated. The table shows that in the combined areas, as also in the quadrilateral, the pure correlation of diarrhoea and dirt was definite in amount in both sets. In the triangle, the pure correlation figure had a minus value, both, however, for size of family and diarrhoea, as well as for diarrhoea and dirt. But we are already prepared for this by having noted the great predominance in this area of that capricious factor discussed in Sect. V, 1 (*f*), which has determined marked irregularity in the distribution of infection throughout this district (cf. p. 49). And it will be shown that in attacked houses there was still a greater incidence within dirty houses. Moreover, it may almost certainly be taken for granted that in normal circumstances there would be a positive correlation between size of the family and diarrhoea, from the greater chance of one out of a large family being attacked, and also from the greater chance therefore of one of a large family being closely associated with a case of diarrhoea: and therefore the minus correlation obtained points to the conclusion that the conditions were quite abnormal. In houses without infants, however, the pure correlation figure for diarrhoea and dirt is much greater, the antagonistic influence of houses containing infants having been eliminated; and this holds for both the triangle and quadrilateral. Finally, whatever the nature of the results in the triangle may be, they cannot nullify the large correlation figures obtained between diarrhoea and dirtiness in the quadrilateral area.

This is perhaps the most appropriate place for the discussion of *the mass action of houses containing infants.* It will have been already noticed that the two areas vary to some extent in the degree with which they exhibit the influences of the various causative factors. Thus, the striking factor in determining the distribution in the quadrilateral is dirtiness, babies being relatively unimportant. The converse of this holds good in the triangle. When, then, the areas were divided up into two classes of sections, containing respectively a high percentage of houses with infants (under 2), and a low percentage, on a similar principle to the division into the high incidence and low incidence sections, it was found that such houses in the high percentage sections of the quadrilateral were only slightly more affected, but in the triangle they were much more frequently attacked than such houses in the low percentage sections, the proportionate incidence of diarrhoea in the combined areas upon the two classes being as 77 : 56. In other words, owing to the mass action of households containing babies, the chance of an infant being attacked with diarrhoea is greatly increased by the fact of its home being closely adjacent to a number of other houses containing infants (cf. also p. 153). Owing to the greater affection of clean houses of this class, no qualification need be made for dirtiness. The high percentage sections were however located in somewhat dirtier neighbourhoods. The different distributions of breast-fed babies account for the differences above noted between the two areas (cf. Table XIX *b*).

(*h*) *The effect of dirtiness in increasing the spread of diarrhoea within the household, amongst the various members of the family.*

From Table XXVIII it is gathered that there is a decidedly greater incidence upon members of the family within dirty households than within clean. This was constantly found in all analyses. The apparently smaller excessive incidence within the dirty houses containing infants than within those not containing infants is evidently related to the peculiarly opposite incidence of the disease upon clean houses of this class. It is not improbable (although there is some doubt as to how these tables should be read) that there is really a greater difference in houses containing infants than in others. This is supported by the fact that there was, notwithstanding the opposite tendency just mentioned, actually a much greater incidence within dirty houses, especially in the triangle—the most irregular area—when only attacked houses containing infants were considered (cf. Table XXVIII *b*). It has already been shown that the presence of babies in a house increases the liability of other members to attack (Table V), but particularly of the parents. Finally, too much must not be expected from comparisons of this kind; as owing to the marked community of infection, exhibited in the clumps, and the fact that most attacked houses of both classes are included in such clumps, it is probable that the chances of infection upon the various members of attacked households are much more equal than would at first appear,

TABLE XXVIII *a*. *The effect of dirtiness in increasing the incidence of diarrhoea* within *the household. The figures denote percentage incidences of attacks upon all persons in certain age-groups in the two districts.*

Both tables are corrected for the disproportionate incidence, and different proportions of individuals present, at ages of greater or less susceptibility: comparison thus can only be legitimately made in one direction, *i.e.*, vertically, the bottom rows of figures having no absolute, but only relative value. Houses in which dirtiness was not registered are not included.

	Houses containing infants (under 2)		Houses not containing infants (under 2)		All Houses	
	"Parents"	All persons over 2 yrs.	"Parents"	All persons over 2 yrs.	"Parents"	All persons over 2 yrs.
All Clean Houses, having dirt indices 1 or 2	15	16	17	14	16	14
All Dirty Houses, having dirt indices 3, 4 or 5	17	17	18	19	18	18

Comparison to be made in a vertical direction only.

TABLE XXVIII *b*. *A comparison between the incidence* upon other members within *Clean and Dirty Households, amongst* attacked houses containing infants (under 2) only. *A number of houses are included here in which dirtiness was not marked till after the season. No difference of any account results from this.*

	Triangular Area		Quadrilateral Area		Both Areas	
	"Parents"	All persons over 2 yrs.	"Parents"	All persons over 2 yrs.	"Parents"	All persons over 2 yrs.
Clean Houses, having dirt indices 1 or 2	15	17	25	30	20	23
Dirty Houses, having dirt indices 3, 4 or 5	24	25	38	28	28	26

Comparison to be made in a vertical direction only.

whether they do or do not contain infants, and with very little reference to the degree of dirtiness. On the other hand, that the greater incidence of dirtier houses is not due merely to association with houses containing infants is evident in Table XXV, where away from the clumps the contrast became much more marked. As regards the incidence in respect to the ages of the parents: in all houses, and in houses containing infants, the parents averaged only about three years older in the dirty houses.

(i) Conclusions as to influence of cleanliness or dirtiness of the household upon diarrhoea incidence.

(1) *The rather small differences in excess of dirtiness of attacked over unattacked houses*, observed in Table XVIII, and elsewhere, may be attributed to:

(*a*) The irregular and opposite relation to dirtiness of houses containing infants, to a great extent masking the differences exhibited amongst houses not containing infants, when all houses are added together (see p. 44 *et seq.*).

(*b*) The smothering of the differential influence of dirtiness in the houses of abnormally high incidence contained within the clumps; as also in the houses of abnormally low incidence situated in the intervening unattacked rows (see p. 46 *et seq.*). Since about 85 % of all attacked houses are situated in these clumps, it is quite to be expected that the differences between the aggregate dirtiness of attacked and unattacked houses, selected in an individual manner, should be exceedingly small; and we must turn rather to the distribution of these clumps, and to a study of the mass action of dirtiness, for a really good demonstration of the differential influence of the latter (cf. also Table XX).

(*c*) The very small actual range of dirtiness found in any one neighbourhood: it was mostly, though not invariably, confined, in any one row of houses, to two or three dirt index figures only. Thus in neighbourhoods of only moderate dirtiness, the indices might vary mostly between 2 and 3, or 2, 3, and 4—which gives a range of only from 40 to 60, or a little more. Thus a difference in dirtiness of 10 may be regarded as considerable.

(2) *On the other hand, no doubt can be entertained as to there being an important relationship between dirtiness of the household and diarrhoea incidence*; whatever the interpretation of that relationship may be. The combined facts of Tables XVIII, XIX, XX, etc., and of the associated text; along with the internal evidence of the effectiveness

of the method employed in gauging and collecting data as to dirtiness and its proved reliability, where such could be tested by general observations, as in the correspondence of dirtiness with the number and ages of the members of a family (cf. p. 42); yield a very formidable array of evidence. The various irregularities met with have, it is hoped, been so far explained as not to appreciably qualify the large mass of positive evidence provided. Moreover, several of the tables are sufficiently convincing of themselves. General impressions are also not without a definite value of their own: thus the writer felt firmly convinced that the distribution of infection throughout the quadrilateral area was above all things determined by the varying degrees of dirtiness in different neighbourhoods. Chart VII, App., shows that the cleanest parts, in σ and τ Streets, were the earliest and at first the most heavily attacked. Infection, which appeared to be of a particularly virulent strain, remained however strictly localized, and tended to disappear early in the season. Towards π Street however, where very dirty and lax habits prevailed, infection, only at first of a moderate degree, continued to hang about, spreading later in a remarkably wholesale manner. The absence in this area of differences in social factors of other kinds has already been commented upon (cf. p. 31).

(3) *Dirtiness probably exerts no more than a moderately powerful influence*: it also appears to be a predisposing influence *of a general kind*: its manifestations are also *subject to the interacting and qualifying effects of other factors*, such as presence of babies, capricious distribution of infection, presence of much susceptible material, etc.; of which the first two at least generally wield a more important influence over diarrhoea prevalence (cf. p. 48). In accordance with the general nature of its influence and the associated qualifying factors, the effects of cleanliness or of dirtiness are best exhibited as a *mass action*; evidenced as an exaggerated incidence upon houses lying well within dirty areas, and an exaggerated immunity upon houses situated well within clean areas (cf. p. 40); and the practical implication of which is that houses situated within dirty areas, whose unexceptionable cleanliness would elsewhere preserve them from attack, are, so to speak, drawn helplessly into the vortex of infection. Proof of this is contained in Table XX *b*, where of the houses with the low indices of 1 and 2, the 94 houses in the "clean sections" had only 39 % attacked, while the 46 in "dirty sections" had 54 % attacked: of more practical importance however is the contrast of the respective percentages where houses without infants are taken alone; this was still more striking, being as 24 : 48.

It is worth noting that the influence of this mass action is exhibited twice over in the tables; thus:

(*a*) In Table XX *b*, any difference in the number attacked from the number of unattacked houses was almost confined to the selected "clean sections," clean and dirty houses being apparently equally attacked in the "dirty sections."

(*b*) The same thing was noted in Table XXIV, with regard to the "low incidence" and "high incidence" sections, respectively.

In (*a*) the explanation is fundamentally the same as that of (*b*). In the former the mass action of dirtiness has induced the presence of a much greater number of clumps; and (*b*) expresses the fact that in these clumps the differential influence of dirt is completely masked or smothered.

(4) *The manner in which dirtiness of the household probably exerts its influence upon diarrhoea.* In the three sets of tables just mentioned, the further important fact is contained, that, where differences in dirtiness of attacked and unattacked houses are observable, as in the "clean sections" or in the total of "all sections," *those differences are confined to the clean end of the table.* There appears to be thus practically no recognizable differential influence exhibited by the higher degrees of dirtiness above 3, *i.e.*, between the indices 3, 4, and 5. From which it may be deduced that the effect of dirtiness is not due to the presence of dirt or dust *per se*, acting for example as the vehicle of an infective organism derived from a ground or personal source, but rather to indirect influences of a general kind, as those exerted by dirtiness of general living in increasing the chances of infection: so that it is *dirtiness* and *not dirt* which is the important matter: and so that, in accordance with the above noted fact, its influence is most effectively displayed in the marked effect of *scrupulous cleanliness* in obstructing the passage of the disease and in warding off attack; while dirty living on the other hand acts simply by allowing the disease unrestrained freedom of spread; dirtiness beyond a certain degree not necessarily further helping the already free course of infection. As regards infection by dirt *per se*, such a possibility is probably limited at least to dirt or dust inoculated with the specific virus; the latter appearing, from the peculiar disposal of cases, to have only a limited and very special distribution, and not to be found in all samples of dirt. Otherwise the correlation of diarrhoea incidence to amount of dirt should be absolute. From the above, it also follows that the influence of dirtiness in any neighbourhood is probably wholly contingent upon the local

presence of infection; a high degree of dirtiness may occur without diarrhoea, where no infection has chanced to be deposited. The evidence of the charts supports this.

If dirtiness in the ways of living is then the really essential point, the question is at once suggested, Dirtiness in what particular respect?

Carelessness as regards specific faecal pollution. Here, the conclusions of the preceding sub-section (cf. Tables XXVIII *a* and *b*), as to the confirmed effects of dirtiness within the household, where babies are present, in spite of the perverse tendency to greater attack noted in the cleaner households of this class, are highly suggestive; attention being at once directed to the constant faecal pollution of the floors and atmosphere of living rooms, and to the frequent exposure of soiled napkins where these are concerned, as discussed later on (p. 60). On the other hand, amongst houses not containing infants under two years, dirtiness led to greater incidence upon the houses as a whole, as well as amongst their inmates. Here, however, it is well to remember the great community of infection exhibited amongst the attacked households of a clump, and the excessive incidence in dirty houses not containing infants may be largely determined by the presence of one or two infants in most of the clumps. Again, the presence of infants is not altogether necessary, as pollution of floors will repeatedly occur with children slightly older, when subject to an attack, and pollution of beds is not at all infrequent up to 14 years of age. Want of attention to the cleanliness of the w.c. must also be of importance, particularly where it is situated inside the house. Thus the question of dirtiness might be held to be wholly a question of carelessness in avoiding contamination from, and in removing the traces of, specific faecal pollution; and there are many good reasons for favouring this view of the case; as direct personal infection might thus be produced; or infection might be conveyed directly, or through fly-carriage, to food. With regard to the latter, the influence **of** dirtiness in the household in attracting and in increasing the pertinacity of flies may prove to be of some importance.

Carelessness as regards exposure of food. Great dirtiness of the household generally went hand in hand with a tendency to leave the whole of the current food supply exposed and uncovered upon the table, at least during the whole daytime, although all the houses contained more or less suitable pantries. Perhaps the milk was less often left exposed than the other food; the necessity for boiling it, and for protecting it to some extent, being a generally favoured precept, although no cover specially suited to the latter purpose was in use amongst the householders. It has already been remarked that in collecting the data special note was taken of this habit of leaving the food about. In probably a large part of the houses indexed as 4 and 5, laxity of this kind existed to a marked degree. Direct contamination of dishes and utensils used for the preparation of food might of course occur in a dirty home from the careless washing and disposal of soiled napkins.

In concluding this section, it must be regretted that there has only been room to set out the leading facts and conclusions upon this subject, and a few scanty tables. As some warrant, however, for the completeness and reliability of the latter, it may be stated that they represent the results of many months of extensive and laborious analyses. Finally, it is hoped that this inquiry will be found to have demonstrated a method of satisfactorily gauging the influence of dirt by means of actual measurements, and in establishing its importance as a factor to be seriously reckoned with in practical hygiene.

2. *Yard paving and drainage.*

In both areas the yard paving was in good repair and was of asphalt, consisting of a wide strip passing all round the backs of the houses, and also along any passage-ways leading from the street front to the back-yards. This was the minimum amount of paving throughout. Where the yards were in common the strip was continuous along the back premises. On both sides of γ Street in the triangle the entire yards were asphalted, in spite of which fact, it may be noted, the incidence on the east side was about the heaviest in the area. Off the asphalt there was generally in both districts a moderate depth of unpaved land, almost without exception occupied by a garden. The yards were free from accumulations of refuse and there was a sufficient supply of ashpits or dust-bins, which were emptied at regular intervals. Although an excellent sanitary procedure, in general, it is interesting to note two ways in which an impervious paving might conceivably encourage diarrhoea prevalence (cf. p. 92). Firstly, amongst dirty and careless people, with their peculiar ability to turn the best sanitary provisions into actual sources of danger, its very imperviousness makes the asphalt a means of holding and preserving infectious faecal matter upon its surface, allowing it to dry, and be scattered as dust. Secondly, apart from the above-noted evidence as to undiminished prevalence, there was an impression received that on a sunny day the warm corners of such yards attracted and became a favourite rallying ground of flies.

3. *Sanitary conveniences and disposal of refuse.*

In the quadrilateral every house was supplied with its own water-closet and round dust receptacle of galvanised iron with removable lid. In the triangle every house had a separate closet, and the same arrangement as that just mentioned existed in the new streets referred to above. In the old streets the old privy-and-ashpit had been in use. The latter had been converted however in most cases, into water-closet or pan (pail) closet, and dry brick ashpit. The exceptions are worth noting and are indicated on the charts. There were three privy-pits still used at Nos. 6 to 10 on the south side of *a* Street, two at 149 to 152 in *κ* Street, three at the bottom of the gardens of the seven houses from 55 onwards in *β* Street, and two at 125 to 127 on the south side of *δ* Street. Conversion into pan closet and brick ashpit had occurred on the east side of *β* Street in Nos. 16, 17, and 18, and in 48 and 49 just opposite, also in houses 23 to 30; and again in *κ* Street from 140 to 145. Scavenging of refuse receptacles and closets was satisfactorily performed.

On proceeding to compare the conditions in the two areas, the remarkable fact is at once apparent that the absence of pails and privies and an exclusive provision of water-closets did not by any means preclude the occurrence of diarrhoea; for in the quadrilateral district where this arrangement exclusively obtained there was an even slightly greater personal incidence of the disease than in the triangle.

In the triangle, the heaviest incidence occurred in two adjacent groups of nine houses on the south corner of *a* and *β* Streets. These were ranged round three privy-pits, and the inmates of the five houses using these privies were attacked a little earlier than those of the other four houses which were supplied with w.c's. Owing to defective divisional railing there was free intercourse between the children of the two yards. The writer's first observations were made here; and the cluster of cases occurring around these privies, combined with what I saw of the children raking over the contents through defective doors by which the privy contents and ashes were removed, and of the diarrhoeal motions largely exposed within, made a very powerful impression upon me that these privies were probably acting as a focus from which infection was perhaps spreading through a considerable area. It will be seen from the charts however that when my observations had been extended so as to embrace the whole triangular district, these impressions had to be considerably modified; for in several other parts cases had been occurring just as early in the season as the first in the above-mentioned focus, and it appeared also to be a matter of indifference whether the houses had water-closets or were otherwise provided.

The next most heavily affected row of houses in the triangle was that along the east side of γ Street; these houses were all provided with water-closets, but the backyards were very narrow, and owing to this the kitchens of the southern half of the row were brought within a few feet of the privy-pits, three in number, belonging to the houses facing β Street. The dividing fence was high, but flies surmounting this, or penetrating through the crevices, might easily succeed in bringing infection. On the other hand cases appeared in three of these houses, in one instance a month before any were said to have occurred in the houses to which the adjacent privies belonged. Exactly the same occurrence was also noted in the following season of 1909; and the flies about the privies on this occasion were swollen with liquid ingesta, but those of the same species inside the attacked houses had shrunken abdomens—a point which may have some significance with regard to the question of the movements of flies. In the northern half of the street the incidence was equally great, though presumably well out of the immediate sphere of influence of any privies whatever. In μ Street and other parts of the district a high prevalence was noted, away from the influence of the privies.

In the quadrilateral there were none but water-closets: there was notwithstanding, a slightly greater prevalence. Just outside the north west corner of the area there was a privy-pit attached to three old stone houses (cf. Chart II) which had occupied the site many years before the adjacent area was laid out for building purposes. It might be suggested that the greater prevalence in that corner of the district was owing to the vicinity of this privy-pit. These three houses were however visited as regularly as the other portions of the district and a special effort made to elicit a history of diarrhoea, but a negative answer, which I believe was to be thoroughly relied upon, was always obtained, although these houses contained many susceptible persons, including two grandparents, and eight children—one ten months old, two sixteen months old, and one two years old. Incidentally the fact that the virulent outbreak at that end of π Street did not succeed in crossing the intervening 30 or 40 yards of open grass land to these susceptible children is also of peculiar interest. Moreover, I felt quite certain that these old cottagers had no communication with the collier population at the end of π Street. No other privies or pail closets existed within several hundred yards of the centre of the district.

With regard to the much debated question of water-carriage versus conservancy systems of disposal of excreta, the subject of household dirtiness again presents itself. As regards any differences observed with respect to the spread of diarrhoea or enteric fever, it is not improbable that the crux of the whole matter lies in the *cleanly working* of the water-closet. In the dirtiest districts, blocking of the outlet with practical conversion of many of the w.c's of a district into so many objectionable pail closets, neglect of flushing, and unnecessary soiling of the basin and of other parts of the structure, are of very frequent occurrence. Again, the *film of faecal matter* that is so commonly found adhering to the basin in dirty houses may possibly present as great an area of infection as the conservancy pan itself to a fly-carrier. With regard to the latter, however, the cooler atmosphere of the water-closet appears to be distinctly repellent to the fly. Moreover, the exposure of diarrhoeal motions in a confined space frequented by all the members of the family in turn must be regarded as a very mischievous feature of the conservancy system (cf. Bruce Low, 1887–8, p. 127 *et seq.*).

Faecal pollution within the household. On the other hand, certain facts will now be mentioned, which are quite outside the question of water-closet versus conservancy pan, but which are probably much more closely connected with the question of faecal infection in diarrhoea. Whatever arrangements may obtain as to the foregoing, there still persist, in most houses of the class met with in the two districts, the same peculiarly lax methods of dealing with the excreta of young children up to the age of three or four years; methods which although unwittingly allowed, from long custom, and though more difficult to remedy, yet deserve to attract the same evil notoriety as that of the old cesspool in the basement. I found that children of this age generally passed their motions within the house, in the presence of other members of the family, and frequently in the room used as kitchen and eating room, or in the scullery which communicated directly with the latter and often led also directly through into the pantry (see Chart III, App.). In the case of infants, the napkins were changed in the same rooms and put to soak in the scullery, not always being completely covered with water, and no disinfectants being as a rule applied to the vessels in which they were washed. When napkins were discontinued the commode chair was used, being usually kept in one of the same two rooms; underneath the chair there was placed a tin receptacle, or a chamber brought only when required from the bedroom. The receptacles were emptied into the w.c. and rinsed with water from the scullery tap where the dishes were also washed. No disinfectants were used afterwards. In a few more careful households however the chair was placed in the w.c. and the child sent there to use it.

In non-diarrhoeal diseases with infective motions, such methods of dealing with the excreta of children within the living rooms and in the presence of the other members of the family would be considered highly dangerous; but when the symptom of diarrhoea is a marked accompaniment of the disease the conditions are many times worse, owing to the loss of voluntary control of defaecation which is so common a feature of the disease in children. Thus the receptacle which had to be brought from the bedroom as often as not was brought too late to prevent the soiling of the floor, the child using the chair without it. Moreover, in bad cases the loss of control was often so great that the diarrhoeal motions would run from the child upon the floor or pavement as it walked about. Soiling of the bed at night was noted as quite common in children up to ten years of age and even above, and it was not unusual to find the whole available bedding of the household in the wash when an outbreak had "gone through" the house. Even with careful mothers, where a baby and one or two young children were affected, gross pollution of the floors and yard paving was often witnessed, the mothers being unable to pay the amount of attention necessary to ensure against such occurrences. It must further be noted that young children old enough to walk are seldom invalided, but are generally able to go about throughout their attack.

In view of all these facts, it is evident, here perhaps even more so than with regard to the successful working of the water-closet, that household cleanliness is a matter of supreme importance; otherwise every part of an attacked household must speedily become saturated with diarrhoea infection. To convey a just idea of the important part undoubtedly played by filthy habits, it may be mentioned that in a number of houses in the dirtiest corners of both districts it was found that young children, and not only those of infant years, were in the habit of frequently depositing their faeces upon the pavement around the house, apparently with the full knowledge of their parents. Next door to such a house in π Street, where most of the children had been attacked, I had the opportunity in 1909 of investigating an outbreak, related in point of time to that in the latter, in a highly intelligent and scrupulously clean family of advanced adult age, who courted a most minute and lengthy inquiry into every relevant detail: association with neighbours, and carelessness with regard to food, could be absolutely excluded. There remained but this one fact: habitual pollution of the pavement of the adjoining house with diarrhoeal motions: the inference as to infection from that source—probably by some carrier agency—could thus be hardly avoided.

To this might be added one more of those actual personal experiences which are altogether unsurpassed for the lasting impression they leave upon the mind of the inquirer. It illustrates the need for readjustment of perspective regarding the relative importance of causes of diarrhoea spread. The investigation of a series of cases was begun by making the usual copious notes as to closet accommodation, drainage, etc. But the inconsequence of the inquiries upon these external matters was only too plainly apparent when I entered the house and saw: A dirty, untidy room: the current food supply exposed upon the table: the mother distracted with an armful of young children—none of whom could have been old enough to use the w.c.: *and a recent diarrhoeal motion lying unheeded on the floor!*

Conclusions. As regards diarrhoea, then, the question of disposal of the excreta is apparently not met, to any extent, by the conversion of privy and pan closets into w.c's.

Considering the wholesale faecal contamination inside the house, mostly by young children who cannot use the conveniences provided for adults, the little extra risk from the exposure of an infected surface at some distance outside the house may not perhaps after all make so much difference.

With regard to diphtheria, Davies found at Bristol that the epidemic was specially located in the outlying newly-built districts, which were specially favoured as residences by the healthy and prosperous young families of the working-class population. The inference being that one might almost traverse a town and be able to point out those parts where diphtheria is most likely to become epidemic. The explanation of this very useful observation is more simple than at first appears: it probably lies in the fact that it is in the houses of this class that young children of susceptible age are most thickly collected. And with regard to diarrhoea also, it was in this same class of house that I found the disease most prevalent; infants and young children being there more common than in the old confined and insanitary dwellings in the centre of the town. I was surprised at not being able to discover in the latter situation, which might be called the slum part of the town, a prevalence as great as that in the two large areas. But the above new property generally includes houses exclusively provided with water-closets and built on the most modern sanitary principles: it thus comes about that the water-closet districts or, again, water-closet towns as a whole, may show, other things being equal, a greater prevalence of diarrhoea than privy and pan closet districts or towns respectively: of which fact, moreover, there is abundant statistical evidence. Thus, of the 14 largest English towns, Liverpool, which has for some years been exclusively provided with water-closets—at least as far back as 1899—had the highest diarrhoea mortality rate for the ten years 1897 –1906; although the 14 large towns included several with an actual preponderance of midden-privies or of pail closets over the number of water-closets[1]. Here it may be that with a large slum population the proportion of deaths to cases may be unusually high or that dirty habits of living have persisted to such an extent as to render the institution of w.c's little improvement upon the old privies. Again, the example of rural districts, upon which as well as upon city conditions the writer can speak from official experience, may be quoted, with their exceedingly low diarrhoea mortality rates, in spite of the intimate and appalling admixture of gaping privy-pits with the small confined dwellings of their villages. This must, again, be largely attributed to the smaller density of the infant population, resulting in part from the lower birth rate, along with the greater cleanliness, particularly as regards care with food, of the agricultural population. With regard to the other side of the question and in relation to enteric fever, Boobbyer (1908) has published for a number of years comparisons as to the relative incidence

[1] A very pointed illustration of this argument has just come under the writer's notice in the current number of the *Lancet* (Sept. 10, 1910, p. 852) with regard to Rhondda Urban District, which is a colliery area with a very high diarrhoea rate. The exceptionally high infantile mortality rate of 190 in the 10 years preceding 1909 is remarked upon: it was 138 for England and Wales. Yet "*for many years past the prevailing system in the Rhondda has been that of water-carriage, and among the 25,000 houses there are only 200 which are not provided with water-closets.*" That is to say, notwithstanding the introduction of the system of water-carriage the *principal* cause of the mortality still remains unrevealed. The question may be asked, Do not the dirty habits of living noted above, particularly amongst colliers, with regard to faecal pollution of the household and carelessness with food and in the management of the w.c., constitute this cause?

at Nottingham upon midden-privies, pail closets, waste-water closets, and water-closets. The respective incidences were roughly 21 : 7 : 4 : 2 during the four years 1905–8.

Comparisons between towns as to the effects of the various systems of disposal of excreta upon diarrhoea prevalence cannnot therefore give reliable results, while the more important factors of density of the infant population, of dirtiness, and of divergent case mortalities, are left out of account; apart from the very minor part the former may really play in faecal infection. But whatever may have been deduced hitherto from comparisons of questionable value, it is impossible to avoid the conclusion, on general principles, that the water-carriage system contributes, *or might be made to do so*, a distinct and necessary sanitary reform.

4. *Stables and Manure Pits. Fly Nuisance.*

The importance of stables depends upon the accompanying accumulations of horse-manure, which furnish the commonest breeding grounds for flies, and upon the reputed association of diarrhoea and the *B. enteritidis sporogenes* with which horse-manure abounds. No systematic fly-counts were made during the season, but many observations were made as to the relative abundance of flies at different times, and as to the presence of collections of refuse, stables, and manure heaps, from which the fly-swarms of the various districts probably emanated. The manure heaps and stables are marked on Charts I, II, and III, App.

In the triangle (Chart I, App.), there was only one manure heap in which the larvae and pupae of the house-fly were discovered. It was at the back of a baker's shop, right against the side fence of No. 84 in γ Street; it swarmed with larvae; fowls however were continually on top feeding upon the latter, and the manure was frequently moved; possibly however a large number of flies were occasionally hatched, as the residents in the houses adjoining complained a good deal of flies, and it will be seen that the two rows adjacent had a very heavy incidence of diarrhoea. They included however some of the dirtiest houses in the district, with a high percentage of infants. No flies appeared to be hatched from the other small heaps of manure behind Nos. 27 and 144, in the stable at the back of 154, nor in the heaps outside the district opposite 142, nor in the stable just mentioned. There was no nearness of stables to account for the high incidence in a and β Streets, or in μ Street.

In the quadrilateral area (Chart II, App.), a milkman's stable was placed against the back wall of No. 205 in σ Street and a swarm of flies was found in the manure heap. The cases became thicker at the end of that street, but this was attributable to the fact that the dirtiness of the people there was very great, in marked contrast to the particularly clean and well-appointed houses of the people further along. This abrupt change in the character of the householders resulted from the fact that it was not so desirable a residential site, being a very noisy corner; there being also two shops adjacent, one of which was a fried fish shop. A stable and small manure heap were also found at the back of No. 156; no fly larvae were found on the two visits made; there was a fairly high incidence of diarrhoea in the houses adjoining, most of which had back yards in common. A large manure heap, *which may have yielded the chief supply of flies to the district*, was situated outside a stable, over the wall from the west ends of σ and τ Streets. A large number of fowls were however always upon it. It will be seen also that the parts of the district nearest had not an unusual incidence of diarrhoea. The houses at the end of π Street which were so heavily attacked, were, again, furthest away from this heap; and indeed from all other stables, whether situated within or without the district; so that in this case there seemed to be no special prevalence of flies to explain the unusual prevalence of diarrhoea.

On a careful review of these facts and a close study of the charts, one important fact was however demonstrated. Whatever evidence was obtained seemed to point to the fact that flies, if they were, after all, more or less necessary agents of the spread of the disease, *did not bring infection with them from the manure heaps where they had been bred*; otherwise, the incidence of diarrhoea would have been greater around the stables or at the points where the swarms of flies entered the districts; *but that they only acted as carriers when*, in the course of their wanderings, *they came across an infected household where they could obtain infected matter to carry.* Cf. also the evidence of the prevalence curves (Sect. VII). It would also be most reasonable to assume that their power of infection is greatest immediately around such an infective focus, the infected matter being there most thickly deposited by the fly; and the evidence adduced hereafter as to the tendency to grouping of infected houses gives support to that assumption.

The far end of π Street, alluded to as the neighbourhood of heaviest incidence, was surrounded on the north and west by open country, with no stables or refuse heaps within a good part of a mile. The houses however showed a greater want of cleanliness than any in the district. It is possible that the greater incidence of diarrhoea upon such dirty houses depends largely upon the special influence that dirtiness exerts in attracting the attention of the flies that pass that way. The fact remains, however, that the high incidence was at least not due to mere nearness of the houses to centres where flies were produced.

This fact was particularly well illustrated in a third small area investigated, which furnished as complete a demonstration of the point as could well be desired (cf. Chart III, App.).

The supply of flies throughout this latter area must have been mainly derived from the far end of ϵ Street, where a large heap of manure, from the livery stables opposite, lay always exposed and full of fly larvae; as there were no other breeding grounds within a considerable distance; and because, from this manure heap the flies could be traced all along ϵ Street in lessening numbers, settled during a cold change upon the door and window frames, the doors opposite the heap being almost black with them at such times. The diarrhoea however had its least incidence upon the houses in ϵ Street, nearest the heap, and most in θ Street, the part farthest away. It was in θ Street, and at the end of η Street adjoining, that the first foci of the disease were established, the flies thus apparently only acting as carriers from the time that they penetrated to and had established their quarters amongst these more distant houses, afterwards spreading infection outwards from this focus. In June and July scattered cases occurred; two out of the only three cases occurring in ϵ Street appearing in the latter month. During the first three weeks of August one of the typical explosive outbreaks occurred in θ and η Streets. During this time however no fresh cases occurred in ϵ Street, from which direction any fresh supplies of flies at this time must have been derived.

It was thought worth while, assuming that the rôle of flies is one of superior importance, to test what effect the aspect of a house had upon its chances of attack from diarrhoea; for the reason that the flies appeared to especially frequent the sunniest side of the house. Since the people in the two large areas, almost without exception, lived mostly in the rear part of the house, where the kitchen and pantry are also situated, it was resolved to test whether houses with their rear part facing the south and west really had more diarrhoea. The proportion affected of such houses was, however, found to be about equal to that of houses with the rear facing the north or east. In the quadrilateral, however, the former group had a slightly higher incidence. The districts are however much too small for testing this point, so many other variables affecting the comparison. If however the rows of houses along κ Street and σ Street, whose very small incidence could be attributed to irregular prominence of causal factors elsewhere not unduly evident, could with fairness be excluded, the proportion affected in the two districts of houses with rears facing south and west would be well above that of those having the other aspect; and indeed even a casual inspection of the charts seems to give one the impression that such houses were excessively affected.

Finally, it may be stated that, with the exception of the observation as to *non-carriage of infection from the flies' breeding ground,* no conclusion of note with regard to the areas examined was arrived at, either for or against the question of fly-carriage. It was often suspected, and in the case of District III it was certain, that *neighbourhoods having a low fly prevalence might be more heavily attacked than those with a very high fly prevalence,* and vice versa. Again, the assumption that has been provisionally made, in the absence of exact knowledge as to the habits and movements of flies, that flies are to be found thickest around their focus of origin and gradually spread out from thence in ever decreasing numbers, was very convincingly upheld in the case of District III. The possibility must not however be lost sight of that it may hereafter be shown that fresh swarms of flies may frequently be blown or become transported, immediately after hatching, *en masse* to considerable distances from their breeding grounds.

The subject of fly-carriage in diarrhoea will be still further developed in two later sections of this paper (see Sects. VII 2 (*c*), p. 107 and VII 3 (*b*), p. 127).

VI. FOOD.

Under this heading all articles of *food* and *drink* are dealt with: special reference is made to the milk-supply, the water supply, and the suggested part played by fruit and other solid foods.

The belief in a causative relation between food and diarrhoea is a very old one, and from various primitive conceptions it has passed through several interesting evolutionary stages, none of which, it is important to note, may yet be said to be completely and finally disposed of. In pre-bacteriological days diarrhoea had come to be attributed to purely physical causes, such as indigestibility of food; and the special incidence upon infants likewise to artificial feeding. But the discovery

5—2

of the bacterial basis of infective disease at once suggested the possibility of food infection. At first, no doubt from the fact that the larger micro-organisms and those producing fermentation were the first to become known, it was suggested that diarrhoea was due simply to ordinary fermentative processes occurring in the food, whether within or without the body. Johnston's conclusions (1878–9, p. 212) furnish an interesting and instructive illustration of this point. He says: "I, therefore, consider that (*a*) diarrhoea, as it affects both adults and infants during the summer months, owes its origin in the great majority of instances to the introduction of minute living organisms (bacteria) into the system by means of air or in food; and (*b*) the disease depends upon putrefactive changes in the bowel contents, which changes are correlative to the development and multiplication of these microscopical organisms."

From the context it is evident that he is here alluding to no one organism in particular, but to the ordinary fermentation-producing organisms in general, of a non-pathogenic type and such as those usually found in sewer gas. Ballard (1887–8), however, ten years later, raised diarrhoea, or rather our conception of it, to the rank of a specific infective disease, limiting the cause to the agency of one specific micro-organism. He still, however, appeared to attach most importance to the fermentative changes in the food, and to the substances so produced, both outside as well as inside the body; thus emphasizing the saprophytic phase of the organism (*ibid.* p. 7). More recently, organisms of a more strictly pathogenic type have been put forward. Following up Ballard's conclusions, later observers searched for an organism leading a largely saprophytic existence and gaining admission to articles of food and drink. For obvious reasons milk in particular fell heavily under suspicion, and an important question arose as to the stage in milk production at which infection occurred. Stress was laid upon the possibility of infection at the farm and during distribution; but lately close attention has been directed to the question of infection occurring after the milk has arrived within the home; such infection being perhaps derived from a personal source. The method by which infection is introduced into the milk or food has been ascribed to general causes, such as conveyance in dust, but recently carriage of infection by flies and inoculation of food by that means has received most attention. Interest had centred, however, at a somewhat earlier date around the question of the peculiar immunity from fatal diarrhoea experienced by infants fed at the breast. Thus Hope (1904, p. 42), in investigating, during the years 1884–6, the circumstances of over 1000 deaths of infants, taken consecutively, had found that during the season the deaths of infants under 3 months of age, amongst those fed on breast milk, were fifteen times less than they were amongst an equal number fed wholly or partially on artificial foods. And this matter will be the first to receive special consideration.

1. *Milk.*

(a) *Human and Cow's Milk in Infant Feeding.*

In Table XXX the methods of feeding young children, in the two districts, under two years are indicated. These were practically restricted to two—breast-feeding and feeding on cow's milk. After about six months of age it was a general custom to supplement either of these foods by crusts from the table, a practice which gradually opened the way for a more varied diet; so that in the second year, even though still on the breast or the bottle, most infants received liberal helpings from the table at which their parents fed.

The articles of food which proved to be of really vital importance with regard to the incidence of diarrhoea were two—*human milk* and *cow's milk*; and these presented remarkably opposite qualities in this respect. The addition to either of these dietaries of crusts or other articles from the table appeared to have no effect, at least up to the ninth month, upon the markedly low incidence of the disease that accompanied the giving of breast milk or upon the very high incidence obtaining where breast milk was replaced by cow's milk.

The percentage incidence of the disease upon the first year where breast milk was given was 32 %, and 90 % in the case of cow's milk; and the younger the child when the substitution for cow's milk took place the more liable did it appear to be to contract diarrhoea. The method of feeding had also a considerable effect upon the duration of attack and the tendency to recurrence in the same season, as shown in the following table, formed upon the data dealt with in Table XXX:

TABLE XXIX.

	Breast milk only	Breast & cow's milk, or crust	Cow's milk, etc.
Average *duration* of illness in days { Under 1 year	8	8	14
1 to 2 years	7	24	11
Percentage having *recurrent* attacks, under 2 years	0	8	15

Epidemic Diarrhoea

This inquiry, then, furnishes an interesting demonstration, and probably one that is unique as regards data obtained in a consecutive manner and relating to diarrhoea sickness, of the fact that the above described low diarrhoeal death rate of breast-fed infants depends, not merely upon the lessened chance of an attack ending fatally, but also to a large extent upon the lessened chance of attack occurring at all.

TABLE XXX. *Showing the method of feeding of 105 children under 2 years in the triangular and quadrilateral areas, and the proportion in each feeding-group affected with diarrhoea. The latter is expressed as a fraction by placing the number attacked over the total number fed in any specified way; the equivalent percentage is also in some cases placed beside the fraction.*

Method of feeding	First year	Second year	(0—3) mths.	(3—6) mths.	(6—9) mths.	(9—12) mths.	(12—15) mths.	(15—18) mths.	(18—21) mths.	(21—24) mths.
			First year				Second year			
Breast milk, wholly or partially	14/46 32	5/12 41	0/11 0	3/11 27	4/15 26	8/9 88	4/6 66	1/2 50	0/2 0	0/2 0
Cow's milk, wholly or partially (but no breast milk)	18/20 90	11/21 61	—	3/3 100	4/4 100	7/9 77	4/8 50	5/7 71	2/3 66	2/3 66
Details of feeding:										
Breast milk only	8/27 29	1/2 50	0/6	2/8	4/7	3/8	1/4	0/1	—	—
Breast milk, crusts, etc. ...	5/16 31	2/6 33	0/2	1/2	1/4	4/4	2	—	0/1	0/1
Breast & Cow's milk, & crusts or farinaceous foods, etc.	2/3 66	2/4 50	—	1/1	0/1	1/1	1/1	1/2	0/1	0/1
Cow's milk only	12/12 100	4/9 44	—	4/4	6/6	3/3	0/2	2/4	—	2/3
Cow's milk & crusts or farinaceous foods, etc.	6/8 75	9/12 75	—	2/2	—	4/5	4/6	3/3	2/3	—
Condensed milk only	0/2 0	—	0/1	—	0/1	—	—	—	—	—
Same food as parents ...	—	4/4 100	—	—	—	—	1/1	2/2	1/1	—
Feeding unrecorded ...	0/2 0	8/15 53	0/1	—	0/1	2/3	2/4	—	4/5	1/3
Totals in both districts ...	33/73 45	30/52 57	0/15 0	9/17 52	8/22 40	15/21 71	11/19 57	8/11 72	7/14 64	3/8 37

Details as to boiling of milk before feeding.

		First year	Second year	(0—3)	(3—6)	(6—9)	(9—12)	(12—15)	(15—18)	(18—21)	(21—24)
Cow's milk wholly or partially (no breast milk)	Boiled	17/18 94	11/16 66	—	3/3	3/3	7/7	4/6	4/4	2/3	1/2
	Unboiled or sometimes so	1/2 50	2/5 50	—	1/1	—	0/1	0/2	2/3	—	1/1
Cow's milk only	Boiled	12/12 100	4/9 42	—	4/4	6/6	3/3	0/2	2/3	—	1/2
	Unboiled or sometimes so	0/2 0	1/2 50	—	—	—	—	—	0/1	—	1/1
Cow's milk and crusts or farinaceous foods	Boiled	6/8 83	7/8 87	—	1/1	—	4/5	4/4	1/1	2/3	—
	Unboiled or sometimes so	1/2 50	2/4 50	—	1/1	—	0/1	0/2	2/3	—	—

As regards the explanation of these facts, it is conceivable that breast milk may act in one or both of two ways: either it plays a passive part, where it is partaken of to the exclusion of all other foods; thus ensuring, firstly, a wholly germ-free diet; and secondly, the exclusion of foreign—and consequently irritant and less nourishing—milks and other foods: or, its rôle is an active one, exercising, by means of certain vital properties, an inhibitive or bactericidal action upon any infective bodies introduced in the food. The cow's milk, again, may act either mechanically, by its irritant action upon digestion, being a foreign milk and to that extent an unnatural food: or specifically, by being the vehicle through which the specific virus is generally introduced into the body. Of course the cow's milk might conceivably produce its effect in both of these ways, the former one paving the way for the latter.

There were two reasons for giving serious consideration to the merely irritative effect of cow's milk upon digestion. The first was that the younger the child, and consequently the more limited and the less adaptable its digestive powers, the greater was the incidence upon those fed on that milk. Under 9 months every child so fed contracted diarrhoea. The second was, that boiling the milk before feeding had no effect in preventing the disease; thus making it difficult to believe at least that the diarrhoea was due to a living and specific infective agent. It is also possible that boiling actually increased the irritant properties of the foreign milk, just as it impairs the properties of the natural milk.

The boiling of milk. Turning to the question of boiling: the results obtained were very remarkable. Boiling appeared to produce no effect at all; or if anything, it appeared to increase the liability to diarrhoea; perhaps in the way suggested above. If however it be supposed that the cause of diarrhoea is generally introduced in milk, and is a living virus, boiling before feeding, even if the routine of feeding is not always in accord with scientifically perfect asepsis, should at least produce *some* decrease in the incidence of diarrhoea. The fact that boiling had no effect may be interpreted in one or more of three ways: either the actual cause of the disease is not affected by boiling—in that case recalling the interesting theories that it may depend simply upon the presence of toxins in milk as a direct or merely predisposing cause, or upon the presence of a sporing organism which can resist the heat: or secondly, it may point to the fact that infection by milk is not really of great importance as a method of spread, that other foods are just as important, or that some other method must be sought, as *e.g.*, that of direct personal infection : or thirdly, the process of boiling may, and probably does, destroy certain vital properties of milk which inhibit the growth of disease organisms, whether or not that protection may depend upon the presence of the inhibitory lactic acid organisms ; or increases, by the chemical changes it induces, the irritant action of a foreign milk.

It will be noticed that in these districts the practice of boiling the milk, before feeding infants under one year, was almost universal ; a practice which was no doubt the good result of the many years of persistent local medical teaching upon the subject. The employment of the modern tubeless feeding bottle was also, for similar reasons, quite the usual practice. Milk partaken of by children, above the age of 2 years, was usually derived from the general household supply, which in summer at least was generally boiled on receipt. In 71 % of 53 houses canvassed it was recorded that the milk was "generally boiled" or "always boiled." At ages 2, 3, and 4, where a mixed diet was partaken of with the addition of drinks of milk, there was some slight indication of a greater incidence with unboiled milk ; but the figures were too small and incomplete—data not being systematically gathered upon this point—to draw reliable conclusions from ; there being only 11 children, at the three ages, recorded as partaking of unboiled milk.

From what has been here put forward as to the boiling of milk, the proffering of advice to the general public to boil their milk in summer would appear to be so much labour in vain, as regards the prevention of diarrhoea. It is important to note however that the evidence obtained as to the ineffectiveness of boiling, as a home procedure amongst an uninstructed public, is not directly antagonistic to the practice of distributing milk, produced, sterilized, and delivered in sealed bottles, from scientifically organised and controlled milk depots ; although the absence of any effect at all in the home treatment of milk rather suggests the inutility of boiling under most circumstances.

The above conclusions might be supported by quotations from several recent papers on this subject (cf. some in the list quoted at the foot of this paper) ; and it may be added that all the possible explanations of the parts played by breast milk, cow's milk, and by boiling, suggested above, have at various times and even up to the present received serious support. Stawell's remarks (1899, pp. 153—7) of 10 years ago have apparently anticipated the present attitude.

Referring to the fact of *stale milk*, i.e., *milk which has lost its first freshness*, being constantly associated with a high diarrhoea incidence, whether it be taken boiled or unboiled, he says "no amount of special care will certainly prevent diarrhoea" with "ordinary bought milk," "even if that milk is pasteurised on delivery." "All bought milk is for practical purposes to be regarded as 'stale milk.'" Upon ordering the keeping of a cow, for the supply of perfectly fresh milk, he was able to bring infant patients through the summer without diarrhoea. The keeping of a goat affords a somewhat more economical means of attaining the same end.

This inquiry as to infant feeding throws a very interesting light upon *questions of age incidence*. It seems that the second year of life shows the greatest attack incidence, but it might be argued that, as in the case of mortality, the first year would exhibit the greatest susceptibility, were it not veiled by the large amount of breast-feeding during that period. Again, the high incidence of the second year may be considered to be abnormally raised by the number of highly susceptible children who have, up to that time, been protected from attack by breast-feeding. These suggestions are in fact borne out by examining the incidence in those fed otherwise than upon the breast, from the earliest months onward. In the second and following trimestra, where artificial feeding has been instituted, the incidence is greatest of all, being 100%; but from that period onwards through the first, second, third, and following years there is a gradual and continual fall.

As regards the rôle of cow's milk (cf. also p. 171), it is a remarkable fact that the rise of diarrhoea incidence to a maximum in the second year with subsequent gradual decline, corresponded exactly with the frequency with which cow's milk appeared in the dietary of children throughout the first few years of life. The most constant article of diet of any one period of childhood is probably cow's milk during the second twelve-monthly period of life. It is the staple article of diet at this time, however varied the method of feeding may be before or afterwards. It was found by special observations that most cow's milk was given at this period, but that it was also given largely, although with gradually decreasing frequency, in the years immediately succeeding this age. Children above two almost invariably partook of an ordinary mixed diet, being fed from the table along with their parents; but according to the tenderness of their years, it was generally the rule to supplement these meals with drinks of milk, as being a natural and even necessary food for children of such an age; the practice being gradually discontinued as they grow up; and it is important to note that the incidence upon the third year was actually as great as that upon the first year of life, viz., 45 % in all houses. These somewhat striking correspondences then suggest the question as to how far the greater susceptibility of certain age-periods is due to the direct effect of cow's milk and the greater frequency with which it enters into the dietary. As the result of a special analysis it was found that the proportion of "first cases" amongst those fed on cow's milk and those fed on the breast was about the same. Thus, setting aside domestic infection for the moment, there was no indication that the cow's milk had played a specially important part, as regards introducing diarrhoea within the household.

As regards the rôle of breast milk. In accepting the simplest hypothesis, that susceptibility to diarrhoea decreases from the earliest months upwards, it is practically implied that breast milk must exercise an active inhibitive influence upon diarrhoea infection. This influence was most marked up till the end of the ninth month, only 18 % so fed being attacked, as against 100 % of those fed on cow's milk without the breast. After that time, probably owing to the impaired quality of the breast milk, the protective influence was largely lost. Disturbances due to teething should be remembered at this period. The large proportion of crusts and scraps from the table that enter into the dietary at this time might also have been held accountable for this sudden change, but that, before the end of the ninth month, the 11 children so fed showed a remarkably low incidence, even less than those said to be wholly breast-fed. From the latter fact it is evident that before this period, at any rate, the notable quantities of household dirt and dust known to be introduced on these crusts appeared to convey no infection, or at least were rendered completely harmless by the admixture with breast milk. Turning to the 22 houses containing breast-fed babies under six months, only three of which babies were affected, it is found that 66 % of such houses were attacked houses. This was a proportionately high figure, since only 70 % of all houses with children under one year were attacked, and the latter include many houses where the infant under one year was the only child affected. The fact that the breast-fed infants remained free in the presence of all this infection (in one case with as many as four other members of the family attacked), is again evidence of the positive inhibitive action of breast milk.

During the season, no cases of diarrhoea were found under three months, but in the November following a typical case was found, seven weeks old, and fed wholly upon the breast. Even at this early age then, there is an appreciable susceptibility, and breast milk is not completely protective against attack. Further than this, five cases, or 20 % of those wholly breast-fed, under nine months, were attacked : in two of these the mother developed diarrhoea one and five days respectively before the child ; but in two others no association with attacked persons could be discovered. Similar results were found amongst children partially breast-fed.

(b) *The Milk-Supply as a suggested source of infection.*

When milk became suspected as a vehicle of infection, one suggestion put forward was that infection generally occurred at some time previous to, or during, the distribution of milk to the householder ; milk thus becoming an important means of *introducing* infection into the home. This view of the case which has always received a great deal of attention will now be discussed in reference to the relations of the milk-supply and diarrhoea prevalence in the triangular and quadrilateral districts. The percentage of attacked households in the round of each milkman is shown in Table XXXI. There were a large number of milkmen, 21 in all, 13 in one district and 15 in the other. Milkmen *D, E, F, G, H, J,* and *K,* delivered milk in both districts. There should thus be ample material provided for demonstrating special infection of particular milk-rounds, should such be at all common in diarrhoea. The comparison instituted, however, yielded no evidence that the attacked households were confined to certain milk-rounds, or that some rounds were very much more affected than others.

In the triangle the four largest milk-rounds, comprising from 9 to 57 customers each, showed a curiously equal incidence upon the houses included in each round, varying only from 50 % to 55 %. In the 9 smaller ones there was a constant tendency to a similarly equal incidence, and the incidence upon all the milk-rounds in the district was 53 %. Again, as regards diarrhoea incidence, the various rounds taken separately were found to vary fairly regularly together with the variations in incidence upon the whole section in which they were contained. The great affection of 9 out of 10 houses in Section I in the round of milkman *A,* might at first appear to implicate the milk-supply, but in Section IV only 1 out of 11 houses were attacked, though supplied with milk from exactly the same source. Absolutely no variation in incidence, therefore, could be set down to the influence of the milk-supply.

In the quadrilateral area, the incidence upon the various milk-rounds appears at first to be rather uneven. It will be seen, however, by consulting the widely differing percentage incidences of diarrhoea upon the various sections of the area, placed at the bottom of each table, that this can be largely referred to the very unequal incidence of the disease upon the different ends of the district, and to the fact that some milk-rounds were mostly limited to one and some to the other end: the incidence of the disease upon the different sections of the triangle was, on the other hand, much more even. In the quadrilateral, for example, the rounds of *R* and *S* are practically limited to Sections III and IV, where the diarrhoea was absent altogether from long rows

TABLE XXXI. *Showing the* proportion of houses attacked *in the* round of each milkseller. *In the fractions the number of houses attacked are placed above the number of all houses—the equivalent percentage being also given in some cases. The districts are divided into sections to afford an opportunity of studying the local distribution.*

Triangular District.

Milkmen or milk-rounds	Houses	Sections of the district					Whole district	Percentages of houses attacked
		I (1-40)	II (41-84)	III (85-130)	IV (131-154)	V (155-184)		
A		$\frac{9}{10}$	$\frac{4}{7}$	$\frac{10}{21}$	$\frac{1}{11}$	$\frac{5}{8}$	$\frac{29}{57}$	51
B		$\frac{7}{15}$	$\frac{7}{12}$	$\frac{1}{3}$	$\frac{0}{2}$	$\frac{6}{12}$	$\frac{21}{42}$	50
C		$\frac{4}{8}$	$\frac{1}{2}$	$\frac{4}{7}$	—	—	$\frac{7}{14}$	50
D		$\frac{0}{3}$	—	—	—	$\frac{5}{6}$	$\frac{5}{9}$	55
4 large Rounds (percentage)		61	57	45	7	61	$\frac{62}{117}$	—
E		—	$\frac{3}{4}$	$\frac{0}{1}$	—	—	$\frac{3}{5}$	—
F		$\frac{1}{1}$	$\frac{0}{1}$	—	—	—	$\frac{1}{2}$	—
G		—	$\frac{4}{4}$	$\frac{0}{1}$	—	—	$\frac{4}{5}$	—
H		—	—	—	—	$\frac{1}{1}$	$\frac{1}{1}$	—
J		—	—	—	—	$\frac{0}{1}$	$\frac{0}{1}$	—
K		—	—	—	—	$\frac{0}{1}$	$\frac{0}{1}$	—
L		—	—	—	—	$\frac{4}{4}$	$\frac{4}{4}$	—
M		$\frac{2}{3}$	—	—	—	—	$\frac{2}{3}$	—
N		$\frac{0}{1}$	—	—	—	—	$\frac{0}{1}$	—
9 small Rounds		66	77	0	—	71	$\frac{15}{23}$	65
Condensed milk		—	$\frac{1}{2}$	$\frac{2}{3}$	—	—	$\frac{3}{5}$	60
Totals of each section		$\frac{22}{36}$	$\frac{32}{52}$	$\frac{18}{40}$	$\frac{1}{15}$	$\frac{21}{33}$	$\frac{80}{150}$	—
Percentage of houses attacked		61	62	44	7	63	—	53

TABLE XXXI (*continued*).

Quadrilateral District.

Milkmen or milk-rounds	Sections of the district				Whole district	Percentages of houses attacked
	Houses I (4-44)	II (45-107)	III (108-130)	IV (131-213)		
P	$\frac{8}{14}$	$\frac{8}{10}$	$\frac{1}{3}$	$\frac{7}{15}$	$\frac{24}{42}$	57
Q	$\frac{5}{7}$	$\frac{6}{10}$	$\frac{3}{9}$	$\frac{9}{22}$	$\frac{23}{48}$	49
P & Q (percentage)	61	70	33	43	$\frac{47}{90}$	52
E	$\frac{2}{2}$	$\frac{2}{8}$	—	$\frac{1}{1}$	$\frac{5}{11}$	45
F	$\frac{3}{7}$	$\frac{4}{11}$	—	$\frac{0}{8}$	$\frac{7}{26}$	27
R	—	—	$\frac{1}{3}$	$\frac{3}{14}$	$\frac{4}{17}$	20
S	—	$\frac{0}{2}$	$\frac{0}{4}$	$\frac{1}{8}$	$\frac{1}{14}$	7
F, R, & S (percentage)	42	56	14	13	$\frac{12}{57}$	21
D	—	$\frac{1}{6}$	—	—	$\frac{1}{6}$	—
G	$\frac{2}{2}$	$\frac{1}{1}$	$\frac{0}{1}$	$\frac{2}{2}$	$\frac{5}{6}$	—
H	$\frac{2}{2}$	$\frac{1}{2}$	—	$\frac{0}{2}$	$\frac{3}{6}$	—
J	$\frac{1}{1}$	—	—	—	$\frac{1}{1}$	—
K	$\frac{3}{3}$	$\frac{0}{2}$	—	$\frac{1}{1}$	$\frac{4}{6}$	—
T	—	—	$\frac{0}{1}$	$\frac{2}{6}$	$\frac{2}{7}$	—
U	$\frac{1}{1}$	—	—	$\frac{1}{1}$	$\frac{2}{2}$	—
W	$\frac{2}{2}$	$\frac{2}{3}$	—	—	$\frac{4}{5}$	—
X	—	$\frac{0}{1}$	—	—	$\frac{0}{1}$	—
9 small Rounds	100	35	0	50	$\frac{22}{41}$	56
Condensed milk	—	$\frac{0}{1}$	$\frac{0}{1}$	—	$\frac{0}{2}$	
Totals of each section	$\frac{29}{41}$	$\frac{35}{80}$	$\frac{5}{23}$	$\frac{27}{80}$	$\frac{86}{199}$	—
Percentage of houses attacked	70	44	22	33	—	43

of houses, and the incidence upon the sections as a whole was very low, obviously from the operation of other factors. The milk-round of *F*, in spite of its low incidence of 27 %, the lowest of any in Section IV, has still the comparatively large number of 7 attacked houses out of 18 in the heavily attacked Sections I and II. Again, the 9 smallest rounds showed a constant tendency to be fairly evenly affected. It thus appears that diarrhoea occurred alike in all milk-rounds, and had little to do with the precise distribution of the various milk supplies. On the other hand, it must be admitted, after making many allowances, that the rounds of *P* and *Q* showed a somewhat constant tendency, even in Section IV, to be somewhat more highly affected than the rounds of

F, R, and *S*; although not more so than the combined totals of the
9 smaller rounds: and it is noteworthy that a careful analysis showed
that this is not satisfactorily explained by differences in the proportion
of dirty houses, or of those sheltering susceptible children contained in
these rounds; although accidental grouping of the customers in peculiarly affected areas will explain a good deal. It is also remarkable
that though the combined diarrhoea incidence on the rounds *P* and *Q*
on the one hand, and that on the rounds *F, R,* and *S,* on the other, are
widely different, yet each of these combined incidences are found to
vary regularly together, in the various sections, with that of each
section of the whole district, as shown at the foot of the table; and also
regularly at all times of the season with the variations in incidence
upon the whole area (cf. also Chart VI, App.). Thus, if the high incidence
on *P* and *Q,* or rather the low incidence on *F, R,* and *S,* had any
significance, it must have been of a constant and general kind, present
throughout the whole season, such as that attributable to different
standards of general cleanliness in the houses of certain milkmen,
differences in the average bacterial content of milk being thereby
produced.

The even distribution of attacks throughout the season has been
illustrated by the construction of Chart VI, App., where the distribution
of attacked persons, as regards date of onset, is shown in the different
milk-rounds through the season. Very complete analysis is given
of the two largest rounds in each district, which were also those falling
most under suspicion for excessive diarrhoea incidence.

The teaching of these charts is particularly emphatic. In both
districts there was not the least evidence of clumping to suggest a run
of cases due to casual admission of infection to a particular milk-
supply; but the cases were scattered throughout the season, the
outline of the curve always tending to conform to the curve for all
cases. Nothing but complete passivity was exhibited in the relation
of the source of the milk-supply to the occurrence of cases. On a
review of the matter, the passivity was exhibited, firstly, in Table XXXI,
in the tendency of all milk-rounds in each large area to receive an
equal share of the total infection; secondly, as regards locality, in the
similarly equal variation of incidence upon the different milk-rounds
with the variation in incidence upon the sections in which they were
contained; thirdly, in point of time, in Chart VI, App., in the even
distribution of cases in each section throughout the season, in passive
conformity to the general seasonal curve of all cases; and lastly, in the

apparent absence of any influence of the milk-supply in determining the formation of the characteristic clumps of attacked houses (cf. Sect. VII, p. 88). Several different milkmen generally served the houses in each clump.

The evidence obtained from these districts suggests then the abandonment of a belief that the cause of diarrhoea is to be attributed to the introduction of infection into the house in the milk-supply, unless it be assumed that cow's milk acts in a general way, and that diarrhoea infection, from some common bacterial contamination occurring during production or storage, is common to all samples of cow's milk. Some milks might of course get more of such pollution than others, and it might be seriously upheld that this is shown in Table XXXI in the quadrilateral area, in the higher incidence upon certain milk-rounds. It must be pointed out, however, that no explanation has been given, in this inquiry as to the milk-supply, of the mass of evidence accumulated under "Epidemiological Features" (Sect. VII, 2 (a)) relating to the characteristic local distribution of diarrhoea, and the evidently purposive grouping of attacks in households which adjoin or have certain peculiarities of age constitution and sanitary condition in common. The mere effect of variation of temperature upon the bacterial content of milk cannot of course explain the latter; and thus, since the main characteristics and cause of the epidemic are developed without relation to the milk-supply, the implication of the latter, even in a general way, seems to have very little to uphold it.

It would of course be contrary to experience to suggest that diarrhoea infection could not be distributed in the milk-supply, or that such does not occasionally happen. A small outbreak in the northern corner of the triangle may have been an example of this. The occurrence of 6 cases in houses 150, 152, 153, and 154, was remarkable from the fact that 5 of them occurred within 7 days of one another, and no others occurred in those houses at any other time of the season, or about the same time in any of their neighbour's. The occupier of house No. 150 was milkman L, who supplied the 4 houses, the only houses— unfortunately for this inquiry—in that milk-round in the district. The milkman L contracted typical diarrhoea and may thus have been a means of infecting the others through the milk-supply. Milkman L did not personally distribute the milk. It was stated, however, that diarrhoea was contracted, in Nos. 153 and 154, four days before the former was attacked. The dates were perhaps rather doubtful, and at that unsatisfactory point the enquiry must be allowed to remain.

Milkmen *A* and *B* also lived in the district, at 142 and 140 respectively ; they appeared not to have had diarrhoea during the season. Due allowance must of course be made for any history of that kind obtained from milksellers. In the quadrilateral one of the milk vendors, milk-man *F*, lived in the district in a house behind No. 205 in σ St., but gave no history of attack in his household.

(c)   *The suggested infection of milk within the home.*

Newsholme (1902 and 1906) at Brighton found that amongst infants dying of epidemic diarrhoea condensed milk was an even more potent source of infection than cow's milk, and that there was also a definite number who developed the disease when fed upon the breast alone. From both these facts he argued that "diarrhoea is mainly due to domestic infection." Sandilands (1906), with data collected at Finsbury, confirmed the two former observations, and also showed experimentally that condensed milk (Nestlé's) not only contained very few bacteria at the time the tin was opened, but that when left exposed to the air at ordinary summer temperatures there was hardly any increase of bacteria at the end of a week; in contrast to the enormous increase occurring in cow's milk, exposed under similar conditions. He suggested that the comparative potency of the two kinds did not therefore depend upon the bacterial content, that is, upon the total number of bacteria they came to contain. Moreover, since from Park (1901) and Delépine's (1903) experiments it might be fairly deduced that the bacterial content and related pathogenicity of milk varies directly with the height of the shade temperature ; and since the number of cases of diarrhoea (mortality) are not found to maintain a constant proportion to the degree of air temperature, particularly when the ends and middle of the epidemic period are compared ; he there-fore concluded, for this reason also, that no direct influence on the incidence of diarrhoea was referable to the mere bacterial content of milk. Various reasons will however be given later (p. 146) why the absence of an absolute numerical relation of cases to the air tempera-ture is not necessarily inconsistent with a direct influence of tem-perature upon the bacterial content of food ; amongst which is included the possibility that the cause of the disease is limited to one specific organism, not of general distribution, whose thorough dissemination at the beginning of the season is a matter of some little time.

As regards the special importance assigned to infection through milk, it can be readily understood how when infection by food came to be accepted the former had the misfortune to fall doubly and possibly unduly under suspicion, from being a medium so eminently suited for the multiplication of bacteria, and also from being so generally distributed as an article of food.

In the districts under consideration a number of inquiries were made as to the amount of milk taken per household, and as to how it was finally disposed of amongst the various members of the family. From this it appeared that amongst the older members of the household, amongst whom the greater part of the total cases occurred, uncooked milk was very seldom taken. The practice of giving drinks of milk, alone or with other food, to the younger children, as before mentioned, was very general; but what afterwards remained over was usually cooked in puddings. In preparing bread-and-milk the latter was as a rule first brought to boiling point. It would thus as a rule have been possible to exclude altogether the influence of unboiled milk, amongst large numbers of attacked adults, but for the practice of taking milk in tea, which was almost general. This question of milk in tea therefore becomes important. It is probable that, at the time the milk is added, the tea is as a rule at 160° F. or a higher temperature. If it should prove then, that this is sufficient to destroy the virus of diarrhoea, it can be confidently affirmed that a large number of adults contracted the disease quite apart from the agency of milk. With regard to young children, the high attack rate observed in those fed on condensed milk has been noted above; and in a former section (p. 75) allusion was made to the 5 infants attacked, or 20 % of those under 9 months old, fed wholly upon the breast; 2 of these being infected from the mother. In both classes of cases infection must have been contracted within the home, and not by introduction through the milk-supply. Cow's milk, moreover, even as a vehicle of domestic infection, can here be altogether excluded. It is worth noting that the large amount of dirt and dust of the household which must have been introduced upon the crusts of certain breast-fed infants, had, at least under 9 months, no deleterious effect. Finally, a good deal of evidence will be given in other sections as to the frequent occurrence of infection within the home, but not necessarily through the agency of milk.

The question of exposure of milk and food within the home is discussed under "Cleanliness of the Household" (Sect. V, 1, p. 56).

(d)   *Some conclusions as to the influence of Milk, and the Milk-Supply.*

Observations.   *Conclusions.*

1. The possible general part played by the milk-supply as suggested by the unexplained greater general incidence upon rounds P and Q in the quadrilateral area (cf. p. 78).

2. The possible dependence of the greater diarrhoea incidence at certain ages upon the extent to which milk enters into the dietary of those ages (cf. p. 73).

    These observations, both of very doubtful value, suggest that if the milk-supply exerts any influence at all in introducing infection, it is mostly of a general kind.

3. The bulk of evidence as to the influence of the milk-supply indicated that the latter took no part in the causation and peculiar distribution of diarrhoea attacks, *e.g.*, in the formation of the "time and place groups" (p. 79); thereby nullifying the importance of this supposed commonest vehicle of infection from an impersonal source (cf. p. 78).

4. Boiling the milk—generally on receipt—did not decrease the incidence of diarrhoea (cf. p. 71).

5. The proportion of "first cases" amongst those fed on the breast or on cow's milk, respectively, was about the same (cf. p. 74).

    The part played by the milk-supply is thus either a negligible or at least a passive one, the milk apparently coming to act merely as a vehicle of domestic infection, just as any other food might do.   The evidence obtained points to the greater part of infection being caught within the home.

6. 20 % of children, wholly breast-fed, were attacked.   40 % of those attacked under 12 months were not having any cow's milk (Table XXX).   Many adults took no milk, or only cooked milk, and yet were attacked (cf. p. 81).

    Plenty of infection therefore occurs within the home when cow's milk is altogether excluded from the dietary.

2. *Water.*

The water supply of the districts was excellent; it was exclusively tap water, laid on to each house from the town's supply. The latter is derived from deep borings in the sandstone, the works being situated in the Sherwood Forest, several miles out of the town. Water is generally excluded as a possible factor in the causation of epidemic diarrhoea where the supply is unexceptionable in source and quality.

3. *Fruit and Solid Foods.*

Fruit, per se, is popularly held to be one of the commonest causes of diarrhoea; a belief which will not however stand the test of more than a superficial enquiry. There are a number of points of difference distinguishing the simple diarrhoea or irritative digestive disturbance following over-indulgence in fruit from epidemic diarrhoea: the absence of clinical signs of a specific affection, and the absence of related specific cases (cf. Sect. III, 1, p. 19): it has also been remarked that the maximum age incidence of epidemic diarrhoea does not correspond at all with the ages at which fruit is mostly eaten: moreover, the seasonal abundances of the common fruits, individually, and even collectively, do not correspond with the seasonal prevalence of diarrhoea. Thus, the first fruit of the season, cheap and plentiful enough for general buying, is strawberries. It was noted that in 1908 these first became generally available about July 1st. At this time diarrhoea had already appeared and commenced to increase in various parts of the town. Plums have always received special notice in this connection; but they did not come into season till several weeks later again; while strawberries were already out of season before the epidemic had reached its height. Any correspondences in the fruit and diarrhoea curves must therefore be referred to the fact that they are both seasonal phenomena, which though mutually unrelated, are referable in common to the influence of the cumulative seasonal temperatures. Nevertheless the fact should not be passed over that digestive disturbance due to over-indulgence in fruit, particularly when unripe or fermenting, may perhaps strongly predispose to specific diarrhoea; and that if left exposed to infection it may, just as any other food, become the means of introducing the disease (cf. also p. 147).

6—2

A matter might be here mentioned, which relates to some extent to the food-supply of the district: enquiries as to diarrhoea were not made in shops, rows of which occupied part of the frontages of the triangular district: apart from other reasons, there was the question as to whether the shopkeepers would be willing to furnish complete or reliable details upon such matters.

If milk be allowed to be frequently a vehicle of the disease, as the result of exposure to infection, the part played by *solid foods* generally must also be allowed to be important, since they are exposed under similar conditions. A great part of solid food is cooked, but so also was a great deal of the milk in the houses examined. In a number of adult cases milk in any form was excluded, except the small amount added to scalding-hot tea. In many of these, as perhaps in most adults, infection if it came by food probably came through some form of solid food. In conclusion it is probable that, apart from its suitability as a nidus for infection, no particular food has more influence than another, except in so far as it is more frequently partaken of, or is perhaps more often taken uncooked or left exposed to infection.

VII. Epidemiological Features.

1. *Introductory: Theories as to causation of Epidemic Diarrhoea.*

In considering the nature, origin, and transmission of epidemic diarrhoea, it is of special interest and also somewhat necessary to note the evolutionary stages by which, as one of the last diseases to do so, it appears to have finally emerged from the nebulous theories of humours and miasmata, which in the evolution of epidemiological beliefs have been replaced in most infective diseases by the demonstration of the contagium vivum, and of its method of transference by direct transmission or by animal and other carriers. As regards *the nature of the disease* (see also pp. 67–8) the present conception of its specific character we owe largely to the monumental labours of Ballard (1887–8), who by demonstrating an extensive pathology and symptomatology laid bare what appear to be the foundations of a typical infective disease. The evidence as to specificity has been very generally accepted, but the solution of the further question involved as to whether two or more diseases are not represented by these diarrhoeas of seasonal epidemic type will probably depend upon the final demonstration as to the precise nature of the ultimate cause. Again, whether or not that cause is bacterial, and whether the bacteria are of a saprophytic or pathogenic type, yet remains to be shown or at least to be indubitably established. In the present paper the older theories of causation as to mechanical or reflex causes or heat *per se* will be regarded as superseded; and it will be assumed that the disease is due to the action of, or to an intoxication connected with the existence of, minute organisms, whether residing within or without the body.

Next, as regards *the source of infection*, a point of some significance is the long retention of theories, embodying or tinged with belief in miasmatic influences, though they have been practically abandoned in other infectious diseases. Undoubtedly the long observed correspondence between prevalence of diarrhoea on the one hand and meteorological conditions and conditions of soil on the other, has been mainly responsible for this. Ballard's researches (1887–8) in this part of the subject were not so complete as those regarding the real nature of the disease, and they happened to be interrupted at a stage when he had arrived at his conception of the dominant influence of the deep (four-foot) earth temperature. Accordingly he came, at that stage of his views, to attach great importance to "emanations" from the ground; and his "practical suggestions to sanitary authorities, based upon the foregoing results of the enquiry as to causation" (*ibid.* p. 7), are specially directed towards the protection of the interior of houses, and of food, the principal vehicle with him of infection, from these "telluric emanations"; or towards lessening their virulence by keeping the soil, by adequate paving and drainage, free from pollution. He therefore urges that "the whole surface of the earth beneath houses should be so effectually and uniformly sealed with impervious material, as to prevent any chance of emanations rising into them from the soil." Thus, with regard to the storage of milk, he says that "the dairy should be similarly protected from the rise of ground air" and that "the practice often adopted of storing milk on the ground floor of a dwelling house or in some underground cellar should be altogether discouraged." There is no doubt that subsequent observers laid undue stress upon the 4-ft. earth temperature theory, for some time unduly confining their investigations to the influence of the ground, although it is but just to Ballard to state that he insisted on his conclusions being regarded as provisional only, holding himself (*ibid.* p. 2) "at liberty in a future report to withdraw or qualify statements made under this heading"; and he appears to have privately expressed a view at another time that the 4-ft. record was merely to be regarded as a register of the accumulated summer temperatures (cf. Parsons, 1910). A general impression has however grown up of late years that the prevalence of diarrhoea has no relation to the movements of the 4-ft. earth temperature, except in so far as both are the effects of some common cause.

In the paper referred to, the writer (1908, pp. 7 and 8) pointed out that, though it was true that the 4-ft. temperature rule could be shown to roughly apply in this country in seasons in which the temperature was still ascending at the moment of the diarrhoeal rise, yet, in seasons where irregular rises and remissions of temperature occurred with the diarrhoea sometimes rising from a falling earth temperature; and in cold seasons, where 56° F. might not be reached; as well as in hot countries, where the 4-ft. temperature does not drop in the winter below 50° F. (cf. Armstrong, 1905); the rule was quite inapplicable. The claim of the latter to special pre-eminence over more superficial temperatures must therefore be clearly forfeited.

On the other hand it was demonstrated that the air temperatures, or superficial earth temperatures, could be shown to be *the really* important temperature influences; for when one or other of these temperatures was taken, it was found that a period furnishing a certain sum of accumulated temperatures always preceded the rise in diarrhoea mortality. And this rule was found to be elastic enough to suit all seasons, including the irregular and abortive types in which the 4-foot temperature rule was found wanting. Thus the raising of the sphere of causative agencies to—at least—*the surface* of the ground was justified. In recent years it has however been suggested that the sphere of causative influences should be still further raised, i.e., *above* the ground: that the effect of temperature (of the air) is produced by causing an increase in the number of flies; and that the latter are secondarily responsible for the rise in diarrhoea; the interval of accumulated temperatures being mainly occupied by the incubation and multiplication of fly-carriers. The possibility of direct infection from person to person is another method of transference that has also received some amount of attention recently.

A further discussion of the practical application to the question of diarrhoea prevalence of the 4-ft. temperature record, and its reputed close relation to the fall as well as to the rise of the epidemic, and to the fly curve, is to be found on pp. 133 and 135.

The most important theories as to the source and method of transmission of the disease may be concisely tabulated as follows:

(1) *Possible Source or Origin of infection.*

(*a*) *From a source outside the human body : an impersonal source :* *e.g.* a saprophytic organism of the soil : the source of supply of causal organisms being not necessarily dependent upon periodic renewal from actual cases of the disease.

(*b*) *From a human or personal source* : the causal agency being always handed on directly or indirectly from a previous case of the disease.

(2) *Possible Methods of Transmission of infection.*

Direct. {
    (i)   Direct personal infection.
    (ii)   Direct infection from an impersonal source, as by dust laden with ground organisms.

Indirect. {
    (iii) Carriage by flies.
    (iv) Carriage by food, drink, or by dust containing infection derived primarily from a human origin.

It is important to note that several or all of the various factors here mentioned might play some part as regards both the source and method of transmission of infection. Thus the causal agency might prove to be derived from both sources (*a*) and (*b*); *e.g.*, if it happened to be a saprophytic but facultatively pathogenic organism. Similarly it might be transmitted in one or all four of the methods above instanced.

These theories will now be successively tested against the evidence of the data gathered in the various districts of the town.

2. *The Evidence as to causation of Epidemic Diarrhoea.*

(*a*) *The Origin of infection from a Human or Personal source.*

It has been suggested that all diarrhoea infection is derived from a human or personal source, being transmitted directly or by means of carrier agencies from case to case, complete continuity of infection being maintained from season to season by the few cases which are habitually found to occur throughout the winter. It would of course be difficult, if not impossible, to completely demonstrate the truth of this theory, for that would necessitate a proof of human origin in practically every case: evidence will however be given that quite a large part of diarrhoea infection owes its origin to passage from person to person.

The following 14 points deal at length with the evidence obtained in the two districts pointing to spread by house-to-house, and by case-to-case, infection. Reference should also be made to p. 115 *et seq.*, where they are briefly set out in tabular form.

(1) *There was a constant tendency for attacked houses to be found gathered together into groups or clumps of neighbouring houses.* This tendency, which has already been shown to appear to a great extent apart from the influences exerted by dirtiness and the presence of infants (cf. Sect. V, 1 (*f*), p. 46), is very evident in the charts of both districts (Charts I and II, App.). In the triangle there were 13 such groups or clumps, where complete rows of from 3 to 7 houses were all attacked. These were separated by correspondingly wide intervals of unaffected rows of houses.

(2) *Again, there was a constant tendency to grouping in point of time.* This should be carefully followed out in Chart VII, App., where all the most remarkable examples of clumping in the two areas are given. It should be noted that in most of these *time* and *place groups*, into which quite three-fourths of all attacked houses are gathered, few if any attacks occurred in the many weeks of the season preceding or following the period specially indicated; also that the period of affection of one small group might be many weeks earlier or later than that of another closely adjacent. Both of these facts emphasize the marked isolation of outbreaks in the respective groups from one another, and by contrast the very close relation in which the individual cases of a group stand to one another. As regards the explanation of this characteristic clumping of attacked houses, the suggestion might be made that it is due to a mere chance distribution; but even on taking the local grouping alone, its peculiarly well-marked character in both districts, along with the other evidence of house-to-house spread to be noted hereafter, considerably minimize the possible sufficiency of such an explanation: when, however, the grouping in point of time, as well as of place, is considered, the evidence for community of infection is quite convincing, and the question of chance is no longer admissible. Such community of infection might of course be interpreted as indicating continuous transmission of infection from one person to another; but possible infection of each person and house in the clump, separately, from a common source, as from a focus of ground infection, must also

receive due consideration. The milk-supply had apparently no influence in determining the formation of these clumps (cf. Sect. VI, 1 (*b*), p. 79). It is not improbable, therefore, that *the phenomena of diarrhoea prevalence are almost wholly concerned with the local evolution of various infective foci*; the disease not being distributed to the population in a general broadcast fashion, as by water, milk, fruit, or food supplies. The exclusion of the latter factors practically leaves us then with but two possible sources of the disease to consider—case-to-case infection, and ground infection.

(3) The distribution of *backyards-in-common* in the two districts is described in detail under "yards-in-common" (Sect. IV, 4), as also other structural matters which tend to bring neighbouring households into close relationship. *Rows of houses with backyards-in-common appeared to be particularly liable to be affected together, or to escape together.* This is most apparent in the triangle, where common back-yards were found throughout. Houses 6 to 40 in *a* and *β* Streets are practically made up of four such rows wholly affected and three wholly unaffected. The same tendency can be followed throughout on the chart in each of the other streets.

Table XXIV shows that in the triangle there were 179 houses having backyards common to two or more houses, there being 50 of such backyards in all, common to from 2 to 15 houses, and averaging nearly 4 houses per common yard. The distribution of attacked and unattacked houses with respect to these yards was very remarkable, being as in Table XXXII below:

TABLE XXXII. (*Further details are given in Table XXIV.*)

Triangular Area.

	Backyards-in-common having the houses—		
	More than half attacked	Half attacked	Less than half attacked
Number of yards	21	9	20
Average number of houses attacked per yard, as a percentage.	77	—	15

Far from there being, upon summing up, an almost equal distribution of affected houses per average yard, there was an average of nearly eight houses out of ten affected in half the yards, while in the other half about eight out of every ten were unaffected. In other words the division into yards had apparently an extremely important influence upon the distribution of infection.

Such a conclusion must have far reaching practical issues; and although the available data are limited in amount, a detailed inquiry is warranted before passing on.

It might be suggested that, given the characteristic alternation of groups of attacked and unattacked houses, apparent also in the quadrilateral notwithstanding the almost complete absence of yards-in-common, the unequal distribution into low and high incidence yards is only the necessary result of a mere chance arrangement: but the question of chance is largely excluded by the fact that the yards are of different lengths; some are just as long as the longest clumps; and there is a distinct tendency for long clumps to be found in long yards and short clumps in short yards. An extension of infection to the house immediately adjacent, in the next yard, occurs in three instances, and to two houses in one other instance; but on taking in these houses or the yards they are contained in, it will be found that the high incidence yards now come to contain the whole of the affected "clumps" of the area; leaving in sharp contrast a series of practically unaffected yards distributed alternately amongst them. While there can be no doubt of the marked limitation of the disease to yards-in-common, it is not so clear as to whether this was not largely due to the fact that the boundaries of these yards determined differences in structure and date of building of the houses; differences in rent (cf. Table XVI), and therefore also in the class of people; in household dirtiness (cf. Table XXVII *b*, App.); and in the numbers of houses containing infants (cf. Charts I and II, App.). Thus of the largest yards containing four or more houses, the 11 largest high incidence yards contained twice as many infants (under 2 years) per yard as the 9 largest low incidence yards. However, four of the first group and three of the second had respectively low and high percentages of infants. Thus in 7 out of the total 20 yards the incidence was determined in direct antagonism to the influence of houses containing infants. Similarly as regards dirtiness, infection frequently failed to cross the yard boundaries into dirty and presumably susceptible yards, *e.g.*, houses 31—35. Low incidence yards whose immunity cannot be accounted for except by the limiting influence of yards include the following houses: Nos. 31—35, 36—38, 64—66, 98—101, 131—135, 136—139, 159—162, 170—177 (these latter have yard entrances separate from the houses at the other end of the yard; an almost complete division should therefore be recognised). The failure to spread between the following is also worthy of note: between Nos. 19—22 and 23, etc.; and 41—45 and 46, etc. On the other hand most of the high incidence yards showed remarkable immunity, but at the same time striking limitation of infection, *e.g.*, the three yards on the east side of γ Street; and notably the yard of Nos. 41—45, where the wholesale involvement of a whole row failed to spread to neighbouring houses, which, though clean, contained numerous susceptible infants. Finally, on even a casual inspection of the charts, the influence of yards, though difficult to express in exact terms, is undoubted; and for further details reference should be made to the data there provided, and also to Table XXIV. It has already been remarked in connection with the latter table that the influence of yards-in-common in the triangle appeared to act even more powerfully in determining the distribution of the disease than the arrangement of houses containing infants or than dirtiness. The material is of course limited in amount, and the conclusions must therefore be accepted in a somewhat tentative manner.

Other details in the arrangement of neighbouring houses having special relation to closeness of human intercourse. The structural arrangements, leading to the formation of a deep recess between the rear parts of successive pairs of adjacent houses has been previously described in detail (see Sect. IV, 4 and Chart III, App.). It might be expected that, owing to the limitations and specially close relationship as regards human intercourse and fly influence so established between each pair of houses, there would be found to be a greater incidence upon pairs of adjacent houses with their rear premises thus turned towards one another into the same recess, than upon pairs of adjacent houses whose rear entrances faced away from one another into two different recesses. To test this matter a tabulation of the houses in both districts was made, first of all as to the number of complete pairs present of houses with rear premises facing one another, and secondly as to the number of complete pairs present with rear premises facing away from one another. The incidence of diarrhoea with these alternative classifications was found to be as follows:

Of 328 houses arranged in complete pairs of adjacent houses with rear premises facing *towards* each other, 94 houses were affected in pairs, and 69 were singly affected.

Of 336 houses, arranged in complete pairs of adjacent houses with rear premises facing *away* from each other, 92 houses were affected in pairs, and 74 were singly affected.

Thus the proportion of houses in the first group affected in pairs was 57·3% of all affected houses in the group, and that in the second group 55·3%; a very insignificant difference when the rather greater number of total houses in pairs in the second group is considered. The corresponding percentages in the triangle were 59·7 and 59·7, and in the quadrilateral 55·1 and 51·6 respectively.

The differences in the distribution of babies in the respective groups could not have affected the results very much; there was no difference in the case of the quadrilateral; and in the two districts combined, the number of houses with infants (under 2) in the doubly affected pairs of the first group were slightly smaller than in those of the second group, the proportion being as 40 : 44; a fact which rather tends to emphasize the difference in favour of extra incidence upon houses with their rear premises turned toward one another.

The smallness of the difference however, found between houses whose relations are qualified in the manner above described, rather detracts from the supposed importance of direct personal infection and fly carriage; unless it be supposed that flies have rather the habit of frequently passing backwards and forwards along extensive terraces than of confining themselves for days together to one kitchen, or between the kitchens of the two houses facing into one recess; or again, that playing together in the common yard of the triangle, or the frequent visiting between neighbours in the quadrilateral, over-rides the importance of mere adjacency of houses or the sharing of the common recess, as regards the question of direct personal transmission.

The apparent limitation of the disease to common backyards may however be interpreted as being opposed to extensive movements of flies; or, on the other hand, as emphasising the importance of direct personal infection, such yards presumably limiting human intercourse much more than the movements of flies.

Two possible explanations of the special importance of common backyards persistently obtrude themselves upon one's notice. Firstly, the constant faecal pollution of the yard surface where there are young children, particularly frequent when they are affected with diarrhoea. The yards in the triangle, at least immediately around the rear premises, were asphalted; and the way in which such impervious pavement, if in the charge of dirty people and if left unswept and unwashed, helps really to conserve infected faecal material and disseminate it as dust, has already been commented upon (see Sect. V, 2, p. 57), as well as the fact of the encouragement its warmth may possibly give to fly-carriers. Secondly, there is the close association, playing together, and constant visiting from door to door, especially of the young children of the yard. In the triangle the common yards, where the high incidence was most striking, had very little depth—or at least this was true of the part to which the children were restricted. The three long yards on the east side of γ Street may be taken as an interesting example. They were only about 12 feet in depth, between the rearmost part of the houses and the high back fence ; and were asphalted throughout. These yards were kept in a dirty state and at practically every visit faecal material was noticed somewhere upon the pavement, the dust of which must therefore have been highly saturated with diarrhoea infection. What more natural then than to expect that, on this account alone, many of the 24 children under five years of age belonging to the 18 houses of the terrace who were constantly playing together in this confined and highly infected space should develop diarrhoea ! Such a degree of pollution with typhoid stools would doubtless be regarded as sufficient cause for a large typhoid outbreak. It is evident then that with regard to yards also, everything depends upon the dirtiness or cleanliness of the people's habits.

Whatever may be the real influence of yards, it is at any rate evident, from the marked clumping of attacked houses, to be found also in the quadrilateral, that this latter characteristic method of distribution of the disease is the feature of prime importance and holds good either in the presence or absence of yards-in-common. It should be noted however that it was perhaps on account of the influence of backyards, as well as of irregularity in response to the differential influences of dirtiness and of babies, that this clumping in time and place was more marked in the triangle than in the quadrilateral ; and again, it may have been on account of the absence of yards-in-common in the latter district, that the dates of the grouped attacks were further apart, as if infection had greater difficulty in passing along between neighbouring houses.

In order to connect up these observations with those of previous sections, it might again be repeated that these time and place groups of attacked houses were generally confined to a row of houses of small extent, and were frequently distinctly marked off from other similar neighbouring groups. Moreover, only on three occasions—in *a* Street, and in π and ρ Streets—did houses on both sides of the street, or rows of houses immediately behind, or otherwise adjacent, appear to be included in the same group. Thus, if fly-carriers are the cause of spread, they appear to ply most of their time between just a few houses ; streets and extensive back gardens both offering considerable obstruction to the spread of the disease.

The general impression gained then from the study of all these facts is that the disease has typically a tendency to distribute itself in a number of scattered foci formed of clumps of adjacent households. Although these groups or clumps are usually rather smartly involved— several houses of a clump being generally invaded within the first two or three days, and the whole outbreak being practically over in two or three weeks (cf. Chart VII, App.)—yet, it is not often that more than from three to eight houses are included, infection creeping outwards from such a focus in a rather forceless way, and being apparently easily obstructed by such natural obstacles as streets or unoccupied spaces. The large number of scattered cases, found in addition to those included in the characteristic clumps, may of course be attributed to actual human convection or to fly-carriage from a distance. It might here be noticed that all that has just been said of both the clumped as well as of scattered distributions might be interpreted as pointing, just as favourably to infection from a ground origin as to infection from a personal origin.

(4)   The manner of the appearance of related cases of diarrhoea is very similar to that observed in scarlet fever and diphtheria ; *the cases not occurring simultaneously, but generally following each other with at least some small interval between,* and not infrequently with intervals of several weeks between each. The marked tendency of the disease to follow a chronic course (Sect. III, 3), and the possible long retention of infection, with recurrence of attack, after apparent recovery (Sect. III, 4), may be here referred to as doubtless explaining the infection of long series of cases not always apparently connected.

The cases then do not occur in crops, as in measles and chicken-pox, except in so far as a sudden rise of temperature following a period of cool weather in the middle of summer will simultaneously bring on a crop of cases in many neighbourhoods where a few smouldering cases have been already established. By contrast with the diseases mentioned above the absence of crops points to an incubation period of short and variable duration ; and again to the derivation of infection, not from a common source, as in the accidental admission of infection into the common milk or food supply, but by successive passage from one individual to another, whether by direct or indirect means.

In the charts, it must be admitted, there are more than a few instances to be seen in which infection was said to have occurred on the same day, in two or more cases, in the same family or in one of the associated groups of families. Exact dates, however, could only be obtained in a minority of the cases. It was customary to put down the same date for cases of which no more definite statement could be obtained than that they occurred " about the same date." The frequency of multiple cases occurring on the same day is therefore overstated. There were however a number of cases, of recent occurrence, where fairly definite dates could be obtained. On extracting all of such cases, it was found that in Chart VII, App., there was only one instance in which more than two cases occurred in the same group on the same day, and 13 other instances in which two cases occurred in the same group on the same day. In five of the latter, the two cases occurred within the same household. The frequency of cases occurring on certain days, *e.g.*, Sundays, Wednesdays and Thursdays, will however be shown to have been overstated. Six out of the above-mentioned 13 instances occurred on Wednesdays and Sundays, and a doubt must therefore be admitted as to whether the true date was always given (cf. p. 139).

Another fact suggesting the passing of infection from case to case as opposed to ground infection, is that in more than half of the time and place groups of Chart VII, infection appeared not to spring up spontaneously, but to be due to sudden dissemination around some antecedent case or cases that had been going on quietly for several weeks preceding.

Again, the time and place groups in Chart VII, just as the individual cases, are seen to be scattered over the whole season ; differing widely in point of time even in adjacent neighbourhoods. Transplantation of infection from a personal source is thus suggested. Reference upon these points should also be made to p. 137 *et seq.*

(5) *On some occasions the epidemic appeared to perambulate a locality*, gradually passing down a row of houses or a street, successively affecting the various houses in its path, and appearing to use up the susceptible material as it proceeded (cf. p. 139 *et seq.* and Charts V and VII, App.). It could not however be proved with certainty that this appearance was not due merely to an accidental successive development in neighbouring foci. Besides this perambulation of streets, there was some appearance of spread of high-grade infection from one large district to another, the main outbursts thus occurring at different times in different districts.

(6) *The groups or clumps of attacked houses were distributed in a somewhat capricious manner*, often without regard to the degree of dirtiness, the numbers of susceptible infants, the degree of immunity, or other factors recognised as largely determining the local incidence of diarrhoea. Such eccentricity of distribution is regarded as particularly

characteristic of an infectious disease, since it must almost certainly be determined by chance transplantation and actual personal conveyance of high-grade infection (cf. pp. 46, 95 and 137).

(7) Infection of a house or group of houses was in some cases traced to the *introduction of the disease by a person who had contracted it in another part of the town.* A good illustration of this was given in the group of houses Nos. 145—7 in the quadrilateral—situated in that block between σ and τ Streets already referred to as consisting almost wholly of four well-marked and distinct groups of affected houses. The first group in this block to be attacked were houses Nos. 145—7. The father in 145 first developed it, having violent diarrhoea and being confined to bed for a fortnight under the doctor's care. His attack was associated with a similar serious outbreak in his father's family, living in another part of the town, where five attacks had occurred and the doctor had been called in; infection of this latter household being again derived from an earlier outbreak amongst neighbours two doors away. The father at 145 had been a frequent visitor to his father's family. His illness was followed by affection of his wife and baby daughter and of his two neighbours' households, Nos. 146 and 147, within the next fortnight. In all, seven individuals were attacked in the three houses mentioned. There can be no reasonable doubt of the connection between the two foci—that around 145 in the quadrilateral and that around the father's house in the other quarter of the town, since the outbreaks occurred in the middle of June, when only scattered cases were as yet to be found over the town, and none had so far occurred in the block between σ and τ Streets. There was not opportunity of tracing out the origin of infection of the other four groups of houses in this block, but the interdependence amongst the individual houses of a group as regards the origin of their infection is nowhere so strongly suggested by the grouping of cases in point of time and place, as here. Infection was introduced into No. 135 by the mother, who frequently nursed her neighbour's child in 134 while suffering from diarrhoea (see p. 101), and apparently by that direct means contracting the disease herself.

(8) *The immediate invasion of a number of new houses* in the quadrilateral, built on clean meadow land and occupied as soon as finished, frequently before the walls were dry, is particularly significant of infection from a personal source, and opposed to a theory of ground infection. Again, a number of persons developed attacks immediately after coming to live in houses within the districts.

(9) *The large amount of multiple infection occurring within the household* has already been discussed in Section II, 1 (*b*). A comparison with the amount of multiple infection occurring in scarlet fever is instructive. While in these diarrhoea data 47 % of all houses had more than one member attacked, only 20 % of households were found to have more than one attacked in the case of scarlet fever, for the five years 1904–8, at Nottingham (Annual Health Reports). It is at least legitimate to deduce from this comparison that the amount of multiple infection in the household in diarrhoea is quite as remarkable, if not more so, than that of diseases in which transference from person to person is the chief means of transmission.

(10) Important statistical evidence has already been produced as to *considerable transmission of infection* to older members, *within the household,* by young persons of a highly susceptible age (cf. Sect. II, 1 (*b*)): also the tendency to spread has been found to be increased within careless and dirty households (cf. Sect. V, 1 (*h*)).

(11) *A masking or smothering of distinctions, due to dirt and to other factors* largely determining the liability to diarrhoea, has been shown to occur *within the clumps* of attacked houses, or in areas of high diarrhoeal incidence. It is not improbable that these differential factors are here overruled by the influences, apparently more powerful at such close range, tending to house-to-house spread (cf. Sect. V, 1 (*f*)). But the possible influence of a focus of ground infection cannot be altogether excluded.

(12) *A very much greater incidence* was found upon all members *within households* situated *in high incidence clumps* or sections, than upon those in low incidence sections (cf. Table XXV). This probably means house-to-house spread.

(13) *The mass influence* exerted by collections of closely adjacent *houses containing infants* (cf. Section V, 1 (*g*), p. 51), in definitely increasing the incidence upon all houses with infants within their neighbourhood, *necessarily points to the passage of infection from house to house, and from case to case.* No other interpretation meets the case.

(14) A large amount of evidence was collected (see Section VII, 2 (*b*) following) as to the frequent occurrence of *cases where it appeared almost absurd to suggest any other method* of transmission than that of *direct personal infection. Winter cases* must almost certainly be of the latter class.

Presuming that infection is generally derived from a personal source, the possible methods of transmission, by direct personal infection, and by fly-carriage, must next be considered.

(b) Transmission by Direct Personal Infection.

While the general question of the communicability of diarrhoea has of recent years come into some prominence—mostly as the result of observations as to multiple infection and from the attempt to link up the fly-carrier theory, the possibility of *direct* communicability, or direct personal infection, has seldom received more than merely tentative notice. Upon a close search of current literature, it was found that when the question of communicability of diarrhoea was mentioned, there was seldom any recognition of the indirect and direct kinds of communicability, or at least any attempt to indicate what kind was meant. This is probably owing to the fact that mere communicability itself was till recently a matter of general doubt.

Johnston (1879, p. 204), however, in quoting his personal experience of infection while examining diarrhoeal stools, along with the observation that amongst 3,318 cases of diarrhoea applying for medical relief at Leicester, 20 % were associated with from 1 to 6 cases in the same house concludes as follows : these facts " have convinced me," he says, " that summer diarrhoea is contagious and that the chief vehicles of the poison in the above instances were the ejecta from the bowels of previously infected persons."

Ballard (1887–8, pp. 7 and 18) makes but very little reference to communicability in diarrhoea, and that in a somewhat tentative manner. He says, " communicability through the medium of the morbid evacuations does not appear to be a character uniformly attaching to the disease." " In proof, however, of the occasional communicability of an [*sic*] epidemic diarrhoea " he refers the reader to four small outbreaks, which he describes as of the class " not distinguishable from epidemic summer diarrhoea " recorded by Dr Bruce Low in the appendices of the Report (*ibid.* p. 127). In referring to such outbreaks he on one occasion uses the expression " directly communicable."

In a preliminary notice, in 1908, as to the results of the present inquiry, the writer (1908) stated that they pointed to the conclusion "that the bulk of cases are caused by case-to-case infection" (*ibid.* p. 17): also, that while " he was not impressed with the all-importance of milk, he did see a great deal of evidence as to the importance of direct personal infection " (*ibid.* p. 56).

Evidence may now be put forward, relating to the question of direct communicability, and illustrating the nature of the observations upon which the possibility of such an occurrence rests. Reference might first be made to certain parallel occurrences observed in both diarrhoea and typhoid fever and pointing to direct transmission of infection. In view of the fact that both these diseases are lodged particulary in the alimentary canal and have numerous other points in common, it is of some importance to note that the belief has gradually come to be adopted in the latter disease that quite an appreciable part of infection is contracted from direct association with the patient himself. Actual personal experiences of typhoid fever, such as those upon which this belief is based, may here be related by the writer, for comparison with similar occurrences to be instanced in the case of diarrhoea. These include instances of the former disease in a non-typhoid ward attacking a patient in the bed adjoining what was afterwards proved to be a case of undoubted typhoid, when contamination of feeding vessels and actual personal contact could be excluded ; as well as attacks of non-typhoid patients in typhoid wards, and attacks of numerous attendant nurses notwithstanding their special training as to how to avoid the risk of infection. Reverting to diarrhoea, the question at once suggests itself, Are not such occurrences strictly comparable to the occasionally reported instances of diarrhoea spreading in an infirmary ward amongst the infant patients ? Another personal recollection may be added, of one of the not infrequent instances of typhoid fever occurring in an attendant whose daily duty it was to empty typhoid pails. Such, again, are almost certainly, exactly analogous to similar recorded instances occurring in diarrhoea. Thus, Bruce Low (1887–8, p. 127 *et seq.*) mentions, for example, in describing the outbreaks discussed further on, several cases in which infection followed upon mere presence in a room where diarrhoeal motions were being passed or had been voided on the floor : Johnston (1879, p. 204) again relates the curious personal experience of being himself attacked on five different occasions within a month and a half, while making a prolonged microscopical study of the faeces of diarrhoea patients.

Turning now to accounts of actual outbreaks of the disease, Bruce Low's (1887–8, p. 127 *et seq.*) records of the four outbreaks referred to above, occurring in small villages of Yorkshire, are well worth reading at length, and must here be briefly quoted. One of these occurred in summer, at the end of August 1886, and was directly traced to infection from a typical case of summer diarrhoea imported from Leeds— "British Cholera," the neighbours said, was then very prevalent in Leeds ; a series of 60 cases followed in the village. The diarrhoea epidemic in Nottingham, during the same season, reached its acme in the middle of September, and reached winter level at the beginning of November. The three other outbreaks occurred in the months of December, February and May; that is in winter or early spring, when the influence of fly-infection, in two at least, could be altogether excluded. There were 180 cases in the four outbreaks and in all four the symptoms were precisely those of typical epidemic diarrhoea and the manner of infection was apparently the same. In a large number of cases it could only be attributed to the person attacked having been present in a room while diarrhoeal motions were being passed. In practically all cases there had been this history, or that of having handled soiled napkins, or of having used a privy after a diarrhoea patient. The attacks generally occurred during the night or day following such exposure to infection.

Similar instances suggesting direct communicability, collected by myself during 1908 and 1909, will now be given. The sixth occurred in the winter, and the influence of flies could be excluded; the others in the diarrhoeal season. When not otherwise stated, it is presumed that food and other common channels of infection could be excluded.

(1) The most remarkable case was where infection spread amongst the five occupants of two railway signal boxes set upon a breezy situation about a mile apart: infection was clearly carried between the boxes by a relieving man, and all five men were attacked; families of men in each box being also subsequently affected. Two of the men were new-comers, and each was attacked within a week of his arrival. There was no community of food or drink; the latter were always brought from home, and were protected up to the moment of eating. There appeared to be apparently no opportunity for fly-infection of the food; and the only reasonable explanation afforded seemed to be their close association in the crammed quarters of the box for ten hours a day, with the constant handling of the same apparatus; or the sharing of the common pan closet which was placed at a distance of about 30 ft. from the box (cf. Bruce Low, 1887–8).

(2) The next is a case of two sisters who went away together on a holiday, one of whom developed diarrhoea immediately after leaving, but the other not for several days after, and therefore most probably not from the original source from which the first sister was infected. It seems most probable that the second sister had the disease passed on to her by the first, who slept with her, or by a friend who was suffering from a severe attack of diarrhoea when she visited her for

a few hours, just 24 hours before her own attack, and by whom she was kissed on leaving.

(3) In a third instance a little girl aged two years was taken in to play, for an hour or two, with a neighbour's baby, who had a severe attack of diarrhoea at the time. This was at 7 p.m. At 3 a.m. next morning she was taken ill with severe diarrhoea which lasted two days, apparently communicating it directly afterwards to several other members of the family, who up till then had not been attacked.

(4) A married woman, who was herself childless, was in the habit of lifting her neighbour's baby over the intervening wall and nursing it. An attack of diarrhoea in the latter was followed, before its cessation, by a typical illness in the former.

(5) A mother was attacked with vomiting and diarrhoea about midnight; and her baby, aet. three months, developed a fatal attack of diarrhoea shortly after midnight of the following day, "dirtying the bed." The child had been taken off the breast two or three weeks before, and put upon barley water and milk, boiled and intelligently prepared with scrupulous care.

(6) An instance of a collier and his working mate contracting diarrhoea, within one or two days of each other, and where there was no community of food, is—at least—somewhat suggestive.

(7) A little girl, aet. 2, was attacked with diarrhoea and vomiting in January, 1909; and the only neighbour, a spinster, aet. 60, had suffered from a similar attack for a few days previously, during which time she had mended and returned a parcel of clothes to the family of F. 2. At the end of a fortnight, the latter family moved to this town, and the baby, F. 4/12, developed a similar attack, her death about two weeks afterwards being certified as due to "Gastro-Enteritis." Case-to-case infection is here undoubted. "Colds" however took a prominent part in each of the three attacks.

(8) The writer had a personal experience of the disease, apparently contracted while making a prolonged investigation into the second of the above recorded instances. Perhaps an hour and a half was spent in the sitting-room: both of the attacked persons above referred to were present, and one of them was still suffering from diarrhoea. No food was taken, and no flies were noticed. Diarrhoea commenced about 30 hours afterwards and continued for 4 days. Although a mild attack, it was interesting to note that apart from its duration and the mucous stools, the settled abdominal pain and accompanying sinking feeling left no doubt as to its specific nature; these were in

marked contrast to the symptoms of several experimental attacks of simple diarrhoea, induced by excessive indulgence in fruit. Home infection could not, with any certainty, be excluded. There was no recollection of a previous attack: but recollections of this disease are seldom reliable (cf. p. 22).

Before proceeding to the discussion of this evidence, it would be well to first define *what is the precise meaning of the term direct personal infection, as used in this paper.* It is of course a very arbitrary term, and both here and as generally used it is made to include all those cases in which infection through the recognizable channels of milk, water, and food supply, obvious gross contamination with infectious matter, and fly-carriage, can be excluded; leaving no assignable cause but the close association in which the person attacked has been with another suffering from the disease. There is, again, no real line of distinction between this and other methods of infection, as long as these two rather essential conditions as to close association with an infected person, and the tendency to invisibility or apparent unexplainableness of action, are fulfilled. Thus, by analogy with typhoid fever, the typically direct method of infection in diarrhoea might be held to be by the intaking of minute infected particles of dust, or spray, arising in the immediate vicinity of an infected person; the latter being derived from the splashings of liquid stools. But infection following actual bodily contact must also certainly be held to be of the direct kind, the infection in this case following directly upon contact through the hands or even through the clothing. Again, even the usually indirect channel—through food—may come to be considered as a direct one, in the case where infection results from coming immediately from attendance upon a patient and sitting down to eat with hands imperfectly freed from all traces of infection. The above are probably the chief methods of direct transmission in both diarrhoea and typhoid fever; the analogy with the latter disease is justified by the large amount of evidence already brought forward as to infection in diarrhoea occurring largely through the stools. It may be objected however that, in both these diseases, except for a few odd cases resulting from careless handling of the stools, there is practically no occurrence of true direct personal infection, but that every case of so-called direct transmission is to be assigned to the commission of some definite sanitary error which has escaped notice, such as laxity in the washing of hands, in the disposal of faecal matter, or in the protection of food from infected dust or from flies. It is of course as easy to make this assertion as it is difficult, or impossible, to dispose of it by satisfactorily excluding all these possible channels of infection. Infection through the hand, however, may be considered in a large number of cases as strictly a direct means of infection; and from the constant communication of hand with mouth, it is doubtful whether, even in scarlet fever—an accepted type of diseases directly transmitted—more infection is not so introduced into the mouth than is inbreathed. Again, in diarrhoea, in view of the very common habit amongst young patients of passing their motions in the living room, and of the incessant pollution of the person, and of the floors, bedding, and clothing, there is, probably, as great a possibility of the inbreathing of infected dust or of minute liquid particles, as in the case of scarlet fever.

There is however no need to further pursue these theoretical considerations. As a matter of fact the whole matter can be completely and clearly put in the following practical question, as applied, *e.g.*, to the risk of infection from an ambulatory case of typhoid fever—Can infection be caught from such an ambulatory case in the ordinary associations of home life, where no specific preventive measures are taken, but where just the usual rules of cleanly living are observed, and apart from infection through fly-carriers or any of the indirect and recognizable channels of infection, such as the milk, food, and water supply? The answer to this query would no doubt be in the affirmative. It is proposed, then, to submit exactly the same question with regard to diarrhoea, and to speak of transmission of the disease, occurring in such circumstances, as direct personal infection.

Certain practical difficulties attend the satisfactory demonstration of direct personal infection: firstly, the demonstration must necessarily be one of an almost purely negative character, resting upon the satisfactory exclusion of all other channels of infection. And secondly, it must be based, apart from cases occurring under medical surveillance in hospitals, upon histories like those given above, gathered under the notoriously difficult and frequently unsatisfactory conditions of house-to-house inquiry. Collected in these circumstances, final proof of direct infection must be looked for rather in the dimensions of the accumulated mass of such instances than in their completeness of detail in individual cases.

Conclusions. The chief conclusions are set out in the following brief paragraphs:

(1) The question first arises, *with regard to the instances of infection recorded above,* **Are** *they all to be properly included as instances*

of direct infection, and of the typical epidemic form of diarrhoea?
Exception might perhaps be taken, upon the latter point, to the
instances described by Bruce Low, on account of their great infective
virulence. There were, however, no essential differences to be found in
the details of the various outbreaks, and one was distinctly traced to an
ordinary typical case of summer diarrhoea. Moreover, the outbreak at
No. 145 in the quadrilateral area, described above (p. 96), appeared to
be just as virulent as any of these, as regards the severity of individual
attack and the thoroughness with which it swept the several households
involved. An analysis of Charts I, II, and VII, App., shows that the
outbreak in the two districts was in great part made up of small
outbreaks or small foci of infection such as the above. Perhaps the only
difference between these and the village outbreaks referred to, lies in
the fact that the latter occurred in a small community where a virulent
local outbreak could show up to the best advantage, display clearly
typical consecutive case-to-case infection, and have the best chance of
preserving its individuality and the sharpness of its boundary from
intercrossings with other centres of infection; whereas, in a large town,
from the early appearance of numerous centres of infection, and from
the constant intercrossings of infected individuals, this individuality and
sharpness of boundary can seldom be made out. The great difference
in virulence of different strains and centres of infection is referred to
later on (p. 137 *et seq.*).

(2) As regards the precise value of the above-recorded instances, as
evidence for the occurrence of an appreciable amount of direct personal
infection, *their value depends very largely upon the frequency with which
such occurrences were met with* in the districts canvassed. A limited
number of them might always be fairly attributed to mere coincidence,
being referred to unrecognised cases of fly-carriage or other indirect
infection. On the other hand, such clearly traced instances as the above
are not met with so frequently as might be imagined, even in diseases
such as scarlet fever and diphtheria, owing to the considerable intervals,
just as in diarrhoea, that frequently separate related multiple cases.
As a matter of fact, after making all allowances, the numbers and
circumstances of the instances of the kind referred to were sufficiently
remarkable to strongly suggest direct communicability. Finally, it is
important to note all the surrounding circumstances of infection in the
above instances; these were so convincing as to make it appear *almost
absurd to seek any other method than that of direct transmission.*

(3) *Fly-carriage is a factor peculiarly difficult to exclude* in a

demonstration of direct personal infection, from the almost complete parallelism of the conditions favourable to both. Both are favoured by closeness of association, but in both, notwithstanding, infection may leap over considerable distances, owing to the peregrinations of the flies, or again of the infected individuals. Both are again almost equally characterised by apparent invisibility and unexplainableness of action. The fly in its ceaseless journeyings to and fro must in the course of the day penetrate to almost every nook and corner of the house, thus establishing, quite unperceived, continual contact between every person and object in the household. Of course, a demonstration adverse to fly-carriage would at once range a huge mass of doubtful cases upon the side of direct personal infection. It is evident from this to how great an extent advance in the knowledge of the disease and in practical preventive measures depends upon the speedy solution of this question of fly-carriage. *In the winter time*, however, flies are necessarily excluded; and from two of Dr Bruce Low's outbreaks, and from several groups of related cases I discovered in the winter of 1908–9, we must conclude that to a certain extent at any rate direct personal infection does undoubtedly occur in diarrhoea.

(4) The evidence as to limitation of infection to *backyards-in-common* (Section IV, 4, and p. 89 *et seq.*) must be held to favour personal infection rather than fly-carriage, as these yards restrict the movements of persons rather than of flies.

(5) Instances such as those mentioned above, where *mothers have contracted the disease from infants* within 24 hours of their soiling the bed, and where *infants have been infected from mothers*, practically preclude the probability in these cases of infection being conveyed by other than direct means.

(6) *The ample opportunity of direct infection occurring from the constantly polluted bedding, floors, and atmosphere of living rooms and bedrooms* has already been referred to (Section V, 1 and 3). The question might be asked of typhoid fever: How could the members of a family expect to escape infection, even in winter when flies were absent, if the whole household were impregnated with typhoid stools in this wholesale manner ?

(7) *As regards the extent to which direct personal infection occurs in diarrhoea* two facts may be held to show that it plays a subordinate part : firstly, there is the very low prevalence in winter time when flies are absent, in some contrast with that found in typhoid fever : it will, however, be suggested later on (p. 148) that this may to some extent be

an exaggerated epidemic effect; and the tendency of diarrhoea to show a marked uprush and subsequently to exhibit intense seasonal exhaustion (cf. Chart B, p. 120, Melb.) must be noted as in strong contrast to the more leisurely rise and continued prevalence of typhoid fever. Secondly, in the data collected, there was an absence of facts suggesting the passage of any great amount of infection between adults at work or amongst school children (Sect. IV, 2 and 3). On the other hand, the great degree of multiple infection commonly met with (Sect. II, 1 (*b*)), much of which might prove to be of the direct kind; and also the facts as to yards-in-common, and as to infection between parents and infants; all suggest, that the occurrence of a definite amount of direct personal infection in diarrhoea of the kind above described should receive due recognition.

(8) Finally, *the behaviour of the disease in the course of direct transmission is probably somewhat similar to that in typhoid fever: i.e.,* where the fine splashings of stools are excluded, the striking distance is not great; it does not fly across air spaces but *tends rather to feel its way along,* chiefly perhaps on hands which have come into contact with the patient or with his stools or soiled napkins; or again, being taken in with food infected, in the course of its preparation, by hands or household utensils similarly polluted[1].

Its infective capabilities are of course largely held in check by the presence of large numbers of relatively immune persons. On the other hand, remarkable differences in infective virulence of different strains are found, just as in scarlet fever, which also, no doubt, in strains of low virulence, feels its way along in some such a manner as diarrhoea. In strains, however, of great virulence, both in the latter disease as well as in the former, the appearance of actual flying across air spaces is presented, so suddenly and directly is the infection transmitted. Such occurrences were noted in Bruce Low's instances, and also in many of the local foci and of the outbreaks in families in the two districts: the groundwork of the epidemic, however, was made up of a great many isolated cases, scattered between the clumps, and apparently almost devoid of infectious qualities.

---

[1] Such a moderate conception of direct communicability in diarrhoea is not at all incompatible with Vincent's experience, "that no infant has ever contracted the disease in the hospital" (Infants', Westminster); where the milk is described as specially protected "from the introduction of infectious matter from the wards," being brought in in separate bottles, stoppered till the moment of feeding. On the other hand, the conclusion deduced that "zymotic enteritis is in no sense of the word an infectious disease" does not receive any real support from such an observation. See references to Vincent (1910, pp. 8 and 9), and Sandilands (1910, p. 108), at the foot of this paper.

In conclusion, it might be stated that anything more than a reserved judgment is hardly warranted upon a question of such immense practical importance till a very considerable amount of evidence has been collected.

The above facts as to the manner of transmission are important from the standpoint of prevention; and in reference to them it might be mentioned that everything points to the probability that the amount of what has been classed as *direct infection within the home can be considerably reduced*, in both typhoid and diarrhoea, *by scrupulous care* of the hands, and by extraordinary precautions as to isolating the patient, and by proper care in the handling of infection dejecta.

(c) *Transmission by Fly-carriers.*

The demonstration by laboratory experiments that flies can carry infective matter of diseases akin to diarrhoea can hardly be regarded as more than the merest preliminary to the determination of the responsibility of flies for the great seasonal outbursts of that disease. An attempt might be made to crystallize the complex issues there involved into the three following practical questions, categorical replies to which might fairly be demanded before the fly-carrier theory can be regarded as completely established:

(1) *Do flies carry* and communicate the infection of epidemic diarrhoea?

(2) *Is any considerable part* of the infection of the seasonal epidemic so carried?

(3) Are flies to be regarded as the *active and necessary cause of the seasonal outburst*?

In putting the last question the influence of various passive factors, such as accumulation of susceptible persons and a certain amount of multiplication of infection in food, are for the moment set aside.

The second question is seen to embrace most considerations of really practical importance. The third is added to cover epidemiological issues. It is generally understood that satisfactory affirmative replies have not yet been given to the second and third questions.

The problem may be approached, in the first place, by means of fly-counts and subsequent comparison of the seasonal curves of fly prevalence and diarrhoea prevalence. Niven (1904–6, 1908–9) and Hamer (1908 –10) provide data comprising eight sets of seasonal curves. The correspondence of these pairs of curves—which was fairly good—is referred to at length at p. **127** *et seq.*

It is well to note that though by such curves correlation may be established between the two phenomena, that does not necessarily mean causation. They may be merely unrelated phenomena referable to a common causal factor, the temperature. Similarly, there is a large amount of evidence of other kinds, as that to be presently dealt with, accumulated around this question, not at all unfavourable to the theory of fly-carriage, but not yielding sufficient warrant for the institution of wholesale preventive measures and the administrative outlay thereby entailed.

Confirmatory evidence therefore, of a directly experimental nature, is clearly demanded; and what appeared to the writer to be the three essential experiments may be outlined as follows:

(1) *A negative experiment*: that households living in houses rendered fly-proof by wire gauze or other means, though surrounded by infection on all sides, do not themselves develop the disease.

(2) *A positive experiment*: that households duly protected against all other chance of infection, and in which flies from infected houses have been liberated, develop abundant diarrhoea.

(3) *A bacteriological test*: that the specific organism can be demonstrated upon flies caught in diarrhoea houses, and also upon those flies which in the second experiment were held to have introduced infection into healthy households.

Though the third test may be at present inapplicable, the first and second should be quite practicable and present no greater difficulties than have been contended with in the case of Malaria and Yellow Fever; and confirmatory evidence yielded by them would give warrant enough for the institution of any practical measures to check the prevalence of flies or of diarrhoea.

The above suggestions are not included here for purely theoretical reasons: having become convinced of the necessity of such crucial tests the writer made some attempt to follow them up by making, during midsummer holidays in 1909, a personal test of the second experiment on two occasions, but without positive results. Batches of flies were caught in two houses in which several members were suffering from diarrhoea: these were allowed to inoculate food in a very thorough manner, but no attack resulted.

Many observations upon flies and fly-prevalence were made in the various districts; those bearing directly upon this inquiry are described in detail in Section V, 4 ; and the conclusions, as to non-carriage of infection from the breeding ground and as to the frequent want of correspondence in different localities between numbers of flies and amount of diarrhoea, are there discussed.

From the immediately preceding sections (Sect. VII, 2 (*a*) and (*b*)) evidence can also be drawn in support of the fly theory.

The large amount of evidence for personal infection, except that supporting only the direct kind, is mostly evidence also for the possibility of fly-carriage. Evidence as to clumping and radial spread from infective foci is specially suggestive, as well as those facts indicating that it is not the person so much as the house that provides the centre of infection. Thus, while not much evidence was collected as to occupational or school infection, community of infection of neighbouring households was constantly noted ; as if an individual was not so likely to prove a source of infection by direct transmission to those he mingles with, away from home, as to the neighbours adjacent to his house, within the precincts of which it must be noted his infectious dejecta are most likely to be deposited.

Some doubtful evidence collected as to houses facing south being more affected, and as to houses with rear premises facing one another not appearing thereby to be more liable to be mutually affected, might in each case be held to support fly-carriage. Attention is specially directed to the complete tabulation of the evidence for fly-carriage, as well as for case-to-case infection on p. 115 *et seq*. The subject of this section is also dealt with in Sects. V, 4 and VII, 3 (*b*) (i) (3).

(*d*) *Origin of infection from, or emanation out of, the Ground.*

In the preceding sections a strong case has been made out for a personal origin of diarrhoea and for the continuity of case-to-case infection from season to season. It will be interesting to bring forward now certain facts which appear to point to a quite opposite conclusion, and which might be held to support a belief in origin of infection from the ground. In the writer's paper (1908), alluded to before, whilst reviewing the cause of the seasonal rise common to all infectious diseases, but expressly disclaiming any attempt to put forward new theories, a conservative effort was made to set forth all those facts which disfavour a too speedy desertion of the older beliefs, such as origin of infection from the soil, for the newer ones of fly-carriage and continuity of personal infection.

Having become disencumbered, as regards the pre-epidemic period, of a necessary belief in the 4-ft. temperature theory in favour of the influence of a period (cf. pp. 86 and 133) of superficial temperature influences, the oft-suggested lodgment of the infection in the dust could come up for consideration; and it was suggested that the term " ground infection " should be substituted for " soil infection " so as to include infection from organisms lying *on* as well as *in* the ground. It was further suggested that infection might perhaps find its chief lodgment in the dust of the household, and that the seasonal rise of the disease was due simply to the maturing of a high degree of infection in such organisms during a period of certain accumulated temperatures, referred to here as the pre-epidemic period. A wider and more subtle conception of a ground origin is thereby provided, and one which is more proof against hostile attack; for the questions of moisture and of multiplication of organisms thereby lose any necessary bearing upon the question; and in view of the shelter, and of the very equable temperature provided within the household, the perplexing questions of maximum and minimum temperatures, and of the disturbing influences of rain and drought upon organisms growing out of doors in the soil, may also be set aside.

The chief argument adduced in support of a ground origin, apart from relations to meteorological and soil conditions of a general kind, was concerned with *the abrupt annual rise* of diarrhoea mortality, related always to the supervention of an extended period of certain definite temperature conditions (see Sect. VII, 3 (*a*), p. 118) external to the body. From the marked abruptness of the rise in diarrhoea, as well as from the apparent accompaniment, as in the seasonal rise of other diseases, of changes in infective and lethal virulence, it might be argued that the epidemic cases are not continuous with, and not always derived by multiplication of, the winter cases. Certain differences may apparently exist in the nature of summer and winter cases: thus, in the year 1905 for London, the percentage of deaths of infants under one year was relatively five times as great amongst the epidemic as amongst the winter cases. On the other hand, it may be perhaps that only a small proportion of the winter deaths represent specific cases out of which the epidemic cases can arise; the abruptness of junction of epidemic and interepidemic curves (see paper 1908, pp. 24 and 25) could be thus explained. Again, in many seasons, where the data are sufficiently massive, slight or minor rises can be seen leading up to the main rise of deaths; and it is possible that these might have been more often noted but for the very imperfect relation known to exist between deaths and cases; the latter fact being held to be chiefly accountable for the very abrupt manner in which an epidemic will arise at the end of, say, a 10 weeks pre-epidemic period at the unfavourable temperature of 55° F. without any apparent signs of slight multiplication of cases leading up to it (cf. Paper 1908, Chart of Blackburn, p. 51). Collections of sickness data, *e.g.*, those of Ballard and those from Mansfield (cf. Sect. VII, p. 122), suggest the gradual multiplication of winter into summer cases perhaps more strongly than the mortality data. Preceding spring and winter cases are discussed below.

Before passing on it may be remarked that the length of the pre-epidemic interval, but not of course the abruptness of the rise, might, as far as present data go, be quite acceptably explained by the fly-carrier theory (cf. p. 133).

With regard to the Mansfield data, it should be noted that not only a sudden but *also a widespread appearance* of the disease occurred throughout the town shortly after the rise to summer temperatures. As a matter of fact a very special enquiry was undertaken with regard to these matters, and observations were made at carefully selected points, evenly distributed in every part of the borough; 15 of these localities were visited, comprising 4 to 20 houses in each. In nine of these areas cases were found to have already occurred during or immediately preceding the week ending June 20th. These nine areas were scattered all over the borough, there being four miles between the most extreme. Thirteen of the 15 localities had one or more cases occurring before June 27th and the remaining two developed cases within a few weeks afterwards. Thus early in the season, then, it was found possible, by house-to-house enquiries, to demonstrate the presence of cases of diarrhoea in every instance, before more than 20 houses had been visited in each case; in other words, the disease was found to have appeared simultaneously on all sides; and already it might be estimated that there were several hundreds of cases in the town. June 13th might be set down as the very earliest date of the commencement of the summer cases, although for about another week and a half the increase was hardly recognizable.

The important question now before us is to decide, *Whence do these ubiquitous foci of infection arise?*

The difficulty experienced, upon enquiring into the history of individual cases, in referring more than a small part of them to a personal source of infection, might be held to favour a ground rather than a personal origin; but other infectious diseases such as scarlet fever, and diphtheria, present as great difficulties in this respect. Again, when the triangular and quadrilateral areas were separately examined, the epidemic was found to start more or less simultaneously in a score or more of isolated foci, scattered all over them, and apparently unrelated as regards their origin (cf. Charts I and II, App.: crosses are placed in the streets opposite houses containing such early cases). On a minute examination of the data as to 19, and 15, of these cases, commencing before July 3, and July 6, in the respective districts, it was found in the first place, that the cases were distributed amongst all ages, and to some extent in proportion to age and susceptibility. "Children" from 5 upwards were however represented in a smaller proportion. In the quadrilateral, "fathers" were curiously prominent; but in the triangle, young children in the second and third years were markedly in excess; and this appeared to be of special significance, as the 34 houses taken together were found to contain children at this age-period half as frequently again as the total attacked houses in the areas, while infants under one and other persons occurred in the usual proportions. Special attention must be called then to *the important part children in the second and third year play in the lighting up of the seasonal epidemic.* It might be presumed indeed that they are the chief means of carrying over infection from the preceding season. Firstly, because children under that age were practically all upon the breast at the end of the last epidemic, and therefore mostly unattacked. Secondly, because children of the second and third year are most subject to attack (cf. Table II), to chronic attacks (cf. Table XII), and to recurrence of attack (cf. Table XIV); and are therefore more likely than those at any other age to have had the disease in the preceding season, and to have retained infection or to have redeveloped an attack. Thirdly, cases of that age were more commonly met with than of other ages during the winter and spring preceding the epidemic of 1908. As regards the latter, histories of 11 cases were obtained of those occurring before June; five of these were of the above-mentioned age; one was under 1 year; and three, who were attacked in April, were fathers. From the latter occurrence, as well as from a consideration of their moderately high susceptibility and tendency to long and recurrent attacks (cf. Tables II, XII, XIV), the fact might again be insisted on that the disease we are dealing with is not an infantile disease, but one in which adults play an important part, in handing on infection as well as in other ways. The other fact must not be forgotten however that young children of the above-mentioned ages still play nevertheless a more important part than adults. Again, persons subject to recurrent attacks were more than twice as numerous as usual. Finally, it could be easily assumed that certain recurrently affected babies were the means of lighting up the outbreak in their own neighbourhood; but, except possibly in a few instances, no certain connection of that kind could be traced, and the bulk of early cases appeared to spring up on all hands in an apparently wholly unconnected manner. It should be noted that the *main* rises in different districts, as will be discussed later, followed the appearance of these first scattered cases at widely different intervals (cf. the widely different dates of *main* rise in the triangle and quadrilateral); nevertheless the appearance of the substratum of scattered cases seemed practically simultaneous throughout the town.

The respective claims of the ground and personal infection theories are exhaustively treated on p. 115 *et seq.*, where the whole of the relevant facts are set out in tabular form. A few only need be specially noted here.

In the first place, the peculiar form of the typical diarrhoea curve, discussed at length on p. 123 *et seq.*, has been noted as affording evidence of case-to-case infection, from the regular manner of its rise. It is not improbable, however, that an epidemic, dependent wholly upon the maturation of infectivity in a ground organism, might present a curve of somewhat similar form. Variations of temperature in the different situations in which the organisms lie, and consequently in the date of completion of the process, and the increasing probabilities of infection with the passage of time, would sufficiently account for this result. As regards this possibility, in the spring of 1908, I made rough counts of the daisies as they appeared in the lawn, and found that in their case also the curve of increase was of regular form and apparently that of some *probability distribution*. Moreover, having reached their maximum prevalence, they appeared to decline while the summer temperatures were still rising, from exhaustion of the function of florification; the latter however continuing, in some slight degree, until the autumn temperatures fell below a certain point. Thus, in all respects, a peculiarly close and interesting parallel with every detail of the explosive rise and subsequent exhaustion of the diarrhoea curve was presented.

Again, although infection may be always derived from a human source, being handed on by chronic cases through the winter, yet there is always the possibility of a revivification of virulence from symbiotic influences exerted by non-specific organisms derived from the ground, which may gain entrance to the body at the beginning of summer, a lighting up of chronic cases or recurrent cases being thereby produced.

The major part of the evidence can be made to fit either theory; thus, the grouping of infected persons and houses in point of time and place may be assigned to infection from a common ground focus. All the facts favouring a personal origin are of course against a ground origin. Of the facts favouring a personal origin one worthy of special note is the occurrence of cases in houses newly built upon clean meadow land (cf. p. 96). It is important to note (cf. Table on p. 115 *et seq.*) that the ground theory is not supported by any other evidence than that of the abrupt rise of the mortality curve, a point which is however of rather doubtful interpretation.

Whatever value may be attached to the arguments of this section the complete demonstration it affords of *the marked endemicity of diarrhoea* must remain as a fact of real practical importance. The truly epidemic diseases, such as small-pox with us, appear to have periods of total disappearance, subsequent epidemic prevalence being generally clearly traceable to spread from locality to locality. Diarrhoea, however, presents exactly opposite characteristics, being apparently the most markedly endemic of all the ordinary infectious diseases. Figuratively speaking, from the facts above presented, it might be said that the whole population of town and country is saturated with diarrhoea infection, which only awaits the appearance of the warm weather to become released on every side with epidemic violence.

(e) *Infection from Dust, Horse-manure, etc.*

Dust has been regarded as a source of infection, being in a manner a vehicle for carrying and depositing organisms, presumably mostly of a saprophytic type, or possibly a specific pathogenic variety, upon milk or food. Of course dust, using the term in a general sense, is too widely distributed in nature to account satisfactorily *per se* for the very particular epidemiological features and peculiar distribution of diarrhoea above set forth. The dust blows upon all houses and people alike, and moreover in a dry spell of winter may be more abundant than in an ordinary summer. Moreover, diarrhoea has been found by several observers to advance most rapidly in still weather; and thus there is very little evidence of dust being a more common vehicle of infection in this than in other infectious diseases.

Horse-manure, containing one of the organisms, the *B. enteritidis sporogenes*, put forward as possibly the specific cause of diarrhoea, might be brought into contact with food as dust from the streets. Again, it is the commonest breeding ground of the fly ; and the suggested connection of flies with diarrhoea also involves the possibility of carriage of infection, perhaps in the form of the particular bacillus above alluded to, or the *B. coli*, or some other organism, from collections of horse-manure, in which the fly most commonly breeds. With regard to this question several observations have been made that diarrhoea displays no greater prevalence around stables than elsewhere, and the writer's observations in 1908 also yield important evidence on this point, as already mentioned (cf. Sect. V, 4).

(*f*) *Milk Infection, Water Infection, Fruit and Food Infection, etc.*

The actual facts bearing on the possibility of infection by these means have already been dealt with under "Food" (Sect. VI). The possible epidemiological relations of diarrhoea to the bacterial content of food are dealt with later (cf. p. 146). It is only necessary to recall here the possibility that food might be infected either from a human or ground source ; and by both the direct method, as by dust from the ground or by human contact, and by the indirect method of fly infection.

(*g*) *Conclusions: the evidence for Personal Infection, Ground Infection, Direct Personal Infection, and Fly-Carriage.*

PERSONAL INFECTION VERSUS GROUND INFECTION.

A.—Evidence supporting a Personal Origin only.

(1) The evidence of yards-in-common (cf. p. 89 *et seq.*).

(2) Possible perambulation of a locality (cf. p. 95).

(3) Possible movement from one large district to another (cf. p. 95). Irregular evolution of epidemic in different districts (cf. p. 137). Irregular development, in point of time, of time and place clumps (cf. p. 88).

(4) Persons traced carrying infection from other parts of the town (cf. p. 96).

(5) Excessive incidence, particularly upon parents, within houses containing infants (cf. Table V).

(6)   The mass influence of collections of houses containing infants (cf. p. 51).

(7)   Spread to houses newly built (cf. p. 96).

(8)   The common occurrence of winter cases (cf. p. 97).

(9)   The numerous instances met with, pointing unmistakably to direct personal infection (cf. Sect. VII, 2 (*b*)).

(10)   Considerations as to frequent faecal pollution of the household (cf. p. 60 *et seq.*).

(11)   The regular form of the rising curve, suggesting case-to-case increase, in geometrical ratio (cf. p. 123 *et seq.*).

(12)   Solitary cases generally precede for some time the outbreaks in the clumps (cf. p. 95).

(13)   The large amount of evidence supporting the fly theory at the same time supports a personal origin of infection (cf. p. 117).

(14)   The absence of any proof *against* a personal origin of infection.

B.—Evidence not unfavourable to either theory, but perhaps favouring a Personal Origin.

(1)   Multiple cases in the family (cf. p. 11).

(2)   Associated persons and houses seldom attacked together, but generally one after the other (cf. p. 94).

(3)   The regular form of the rising curve, suggesting case-to-case increase, in geometrical ratio (cf. p. 123 *et seq.*).

(4)   The presence of possible connecting cases through the winter, and the large proportion of persons chronically and recurrently affected at the beginning of the season (cf. p. 112).

(5)   The much higher incidence upon the members of attacked households in the high incidence clumps or sections, than in the low incidence sections (cf Table XXV).

(6)   The smothering of the differential influence of dirtiness in the clumps (cf. p. 46 *et seq.*).

(7)   Excessive incidence within dirty families (cf. p. 51 *et seq.*).

(8)   The general influence of dirtiness in increasing the liability of houses to attack (cf. Sect. V, 1).

(9)*   No excessive incidence around stables: this suggests that flies obtain infection from a personal source (cf. Sect. V, 4).

(10)*   Variations of prevalence with variations of temperature (cf. p. 122 *et seq.* and p. 139 *et seq.*).

* ((9) and (10) are contingent upon the fly theory being proved.)

C.—Evidence not unfavourable to either theory.

(1) Clumping of houses in point of place (cf. p. 88 *et seq.* and Chart VII).

(2) Clumping of houses in point of time (cf. p. 88 *et seq.* and Chart VII).

(3) Clumping of persons, *i.e.*, multiple cases in the family (cf. p. 11).

(4) The important part played by the household as a whole ; suggesting that the house, and not the person, is the centre of infection (cf. p. 109).

D.—Evidence not unfavourable to either theory, but perhaps favouring a Ground Origin.

(1) The apparently simultaneous and wide-spread appearance of infection at the beginning of the season (cf. Sect. VII, 2 (*d*)).

(2)* The pre-epidemic interval of certain accumulated temperature influences, without the body (cf. Sect. VII, 3 (*a*)).

(3)* The very low level of winter cases (cf. Chart B, p. 120).

* ((2) and (3) are contingent upon the fly theory remaining unproved.)

E.—Evidence supporting a Ground Origin only.

(1) The abrupt rise of the epidemic mortality curve from the inter-epidemic curve (cf. Sect. VII, 2 (*d*)).

N.B.—Where, in the above, the classification is doubtful, inclusion of the same item of evidence in two groups has sometimes been resorted to.

FLY-CARRIAGE AND DIRECT PERSONAL INFECTION.

A.—Evidence specially favouring Fly-Carriage.

(1) The low level of the winter cases—in the absence of flies (cf. Chart B, p. 120).

(2) The facts suggesting that the house, and not the individual, is the centre of infection (cf. p. 109).

(3) The sudden outbreak in a clump, supervening upon solitary preceding cases, suggests that flies have suddenly gained access to infection (cf. p. 95).

(4) The fact that within the clump infection appears to some extent to rain down equally upon all persons and houses included, suggests systematic dissemination by flies (cf. p. 55 and p. 46 *et seq.*).

(5) Variations of prevalence with variations of temperature (cf. p. 122 *et seq.* and p. 139 *et seq.*).

(6) The almost identical temperature limitations of fly and diarrhoea prevalences, as regards their rise and fall : the significant immobility of the diarrhoea curve till the first fortnight of favourable fly temperatures has passed by : the parallel with cholera (cf. p. 127 *et seq.*).

(7) The correlation of the fly and diarrhoea curves is such as to be quite compatible with a theory of causal connection between flies and diarrhoea (cf. p. 127 *et seq.*).

(8) The large amount of evidence for a personal origin of infection, excepting some mentioned below, is mostly evidence also for fly-carriage (see above).

(9) No real evidence has been produced *against* the fly theory.

B.—Evidence specially favouring Direct Personal Infection.

(1) Continued occurrence of cases during the winter time, when flies are absent : the low level maintained is perhaps against direct methods playing a large part in infection (cf. Chart B, p. 120, and p. 101).

(2) Instances where it seems almost absurd to entertain the possibility of any other mode of infection (cf. Sect. VII, 2 (*b*)).

(3) Instances of infection from babies to parents, and *vice versa* (cf. p. 101).

(4) Considerations as to frequent faecal pollution of the household (cf. p. 60).

(5) The evidence of yards-in-common (cf. p. 89 *et seq.*).

(6) Most of the evidence for a personal origin of infection (see above) might be held to be not unfavourable to direct personal infection.

3. *Some Factors Governing Epidemic Prevalence of Diarrhoea.*

(*a*) *Influences determining the Rise of the Seasonal Epidemic Curve.*

(i) *Temperature and the rise of Diarrhoea Mortality.*

The relations of epidemic diarrhoea to the temperature were dealt with at some length in my paper "Season and Disease, etc." (1908), but almost wholly as regards data derived from the mortality returns.

It was found for Nottingham, London, and most large cities of the United Kingdom, that after the arrival, and continuance, without intermission, of the mean air temperature at 60° F. for a period of four or five weeks, the *main* seasonal rise of diarrhoea mortality took place. The last fortnight or ten days of the period corresponds to the average duration of fatal attacks ; leaving an interval of about three weeks before the main series of fatal attacks commence. At lower temperatures, or when remissions occur, this interval is proportionately extended until the required sum of accumulated temperatures is complete. Thus, at the relatively very unfavourable temperature of 55° F., below which only a very slight and rapidly diminishing influence appears to be exerted, the whole period may occupy as much as ten weeks.

On the other hand the potency of temperatures appears to increase for some distance above 60° F.

The tendency to abruptness of rise of the mortality from the winter level has already been discussed (cf. Sect. VII, 2 (*d*)).

A general conclusion from the examination of several hundred charts is that, upon a rise to favourable mean air temperatures of 60° F., or a little below, there is : firstly, an interval of two weeks, during which no increase of diarrhoea cases occurs, or four weeks in the case of deaths : afterwards, a slight rise occurs ; but an additional period of one to two weeks, or a little more, may elapse before what has been alluded to as the *main* rise occurs (cf. Chart B, p. 120). The period extending from the arrival at temperatures exerting any influence at all upon the rise of diarrhoea, up to the moment of the *main* rise, is referred to in this and the former paper as the "pre-epidemic" period.

In proceeding to the examination of the mortality curve, it is important to note the very strict limitations of the mortality data of diarrhoea, as a gauge, or as a reliable representation in miniature, of the course of the total prevalence of all cases of the disease ; particularly as regards comparisons of different towns. Firstly, the deaths comprise only a very small fraction of all cases and therefore may chance to fall very irregularly with relation to the curve of all cases. Secondly, they are limited in greater part to infants under one year. Thirdly, in deaths of the latter class, moreover, a fatal termination is largely if not mostly decided by circumstances of previous health and social environment : and fourthly, these last-mentioned factors differ markedly in different towns. For these and other reasons, the principles to be laid down in the present and following sections, as to the effect of temperature upon the mortality curve, cannot be suitably demonstrated except in towns

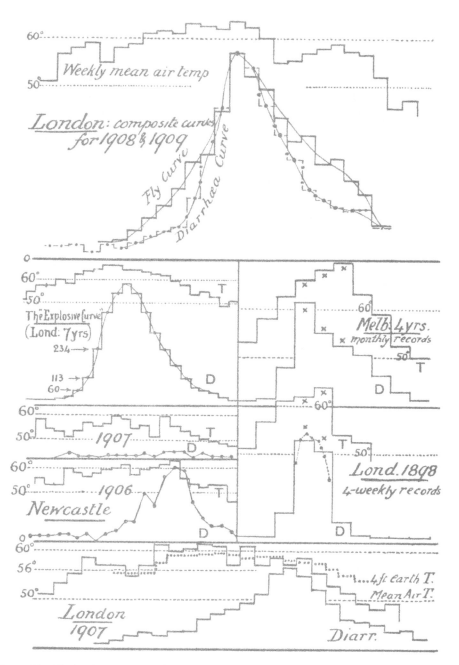

CHART B. Illustrating the typically explosive form of the diarrhoea epidemic curve (Lond. 7 years); epidemic decline in spite of a continuing high temperature (Melb. and Lond. 1898); the inhibition of the epidemic rise by unfavourable temperatures (Newcastle); various peculiar relations to air and 4-ft. temperatures in irregular seasons (Lond. 1907); the interrelations of the curves of fly and diarrhoea prevalence (Lond. 1908 and 1909), etc. (See Explanatory Notes on p. 121.)

CHART B.—*Explanatory Notes.*

N.B.—Weekly records are used throughout the charts, except where otherwise stated.

The Diarrhoea records (D.) are all Mortality data (Registrar-General), but all being moved two week-intervals to the left, they represent Onsets of Fatal Attacks. Mean Air Temperatures (T.) are used throughout (Greenwich for London).

London: composite curves of temp., diarrhoea, and fly prevalence, for *1908 and 1909* (*e.g.* the week at summit represents the sum or average of the weeks ending August 15 and 14, in the respective years). The weekly records of fly prevalence are used by kind permission of Dr Hamer (1908–10). In drawing the thin line a little free, but quite legitimate, smoothing of the fly curve has been practised. The scale of the two curves is so arranged that the apices of the fly and diarrhoea curves coincide: the amount of divergence of the slopes of the two curves from one another provides then to some extent *a graphic representation of the difference in the respective methods of increase, or decrease, of flies and of diarrhoea cases* (cf. p. 128).

The "Explosive Curve": London, seven years' composite curves of temp. and diarrhoea (1897–1906, less the three irregular years 1900, 1902, and 1903). The curve is of the graceful and very regular explosive form, and the increase of cases in geometrical ratio is illustrated in the first part of the ascent where the total of deaths is approximately doubled from week to week.

Melbourne: four years' composite curves of temp. and diarrhoea mortality (1894–8), Dr R. R. Stawell (1899): and *London, 1898.* Monthly or four-weekly records are used. These charts show epidemic exhaustion occurring respectively two months and one month before the decline of temperature: the rounded explosive summit of the London curve and its subsequent excessively abrupt fall, both bear testimony to the fact that epidemic exhaustion was becoming decidedly marked in degree just before the temperature fell. Note in both countries that the same period, two months, was taken in reaching the acme; also the similar temperature limitations.

Newcastle, 1907 and 1906. Showing the power to completely inhibit epidemic rise possessed by unfavourable temperatures. The diarrhoea curve for 1907 became almost a straight line; on the other hand that for 1906, drawn to the same scale, showed that there were local possibilities of a huge epidemic rise when temperatures were favourable. On two occasions in 1907 the pre-epidemic conditions appeared to be almost fulfilled when the supervention of a lengthy and continuous fall of temperature inhibited epidemic increase.

London, 1907. Note, in this irregular year, the failure of the 56° 4-ft. temperature rule; the rise of cases against a falling temperature; the relatively meagre proportions of the epidemic (less than half the average number of cases) owing to rise from a low temperature-plateau; the tailing out of the curve with the lingering of the temperature for some weeks just below 50° F.

Throughout the above charts the temperature conditions of the pre-epidemic period are well illustrated, as also the limiting influence of temperatures at or about 50° F. No very good examples of temperature notching of the diarrhoea curve are however included. A much more complete selection of charts is available in the writer's previous paper (1908).

with populations well over 100,000 ; in fact the effects upon prevalence, and the inherent qualities of the curve discussed later, only constantly emerge in massive statistical data, such as London alone presents.

(ii) *Temperature, and the rise of Diarrhoea Sickness.*

Unfortunately data as to non-fatal as well as fatal cases of diarrhoea are still very scarce. Those that are available however appear to bear out the above conclusions as to the lapse of the equivalent of about a fortnight at 60° F., of the air temperature, before any epidemic cases of sickness begin to occur. A comparison of Ballard's (1887–8, Chart V) returns of diarrhoea sickness, taken from the Poor Law practice at Islington for the ten years 1857–66, with the temperature at Greenwich, supports this conclusion ; as also the sickness data obtained at Mansfield. Chart IV, App., sets out the latter data. It shows that the temperature, after remaining at 60° F. for only a week, fell considerably, and the pre-epidemic period was somewhat lengthened thereby ; the rise occurred in strict accordance, however, with the rules above laid down (cf. also Sect. VII, 2 (*d*)).

(*b*) *Influences determining the Precise Outline of the Seasonal Epidemic Curve.*

(i) *Firstly, as regards the Mortality Curve.*

(1) *Temperature: limiting the extent of the epidemic mortality curve, and producing irregularities in its outline.*

These matters were also inquired into in the paper (1908) above referred to ; although it is regretted that, owing to pressure of space, the reasoned demonstration from the charts was so prejudicially curtailed. It is practically essential to the full appreciation of this inquiry into the phenomena of the epidemic curve, that the details should be carefully followed out upon those charts, only a few of which (cf. Chart B, p. 120) could be reproduced in the present paper. Reasons have already been given (p. 119) why not too much must be expected of the mortality curve in these matters. In addition, in the present instance, the irregular evolution in different districts must be considered : thus a temperature notch may happen to be filled up by a large local explosion (cf. p. 137 *et seq.*) when the data are not massive.

Briefly, *the influence of temperature* upon the seasonal epidemicity of diarrhoea *is, in a sense, an all-powerful one*; *i.e.*, to the extent—as far as conditions in this country are concerned—that, firstly, it is absolutely necessary to the very appearance of the epidemic; failure of the summer temperatures to reach a certain height for a certain time will inhibit its appearance altogether, as not infrequently happens in elevated or northerly towns (cf. the season of 1907, in Edinburgh, Glasgow, and Newcastle (Chart B), with other years). Secondly, it unfailingly brings the epidemic mortality to a standstill a fortnight after the weekly air temperatures have passed, in a decided way, below 50° F. Thirdly, between these two terminal points of the mortality curve it keeps a tight hold of the epidemic prevalence, producing notchings ten days to a fortnight after the temperature variations. Its grip is in fact always apparent; although in accordance with the explosive nature of the curve, the latter rises sometimes with a falling temperature, and so appears to contradict the above statement. In such a case, careful measurement will always show that temperature, as a constant depressing force, has really had a definite effect by slowing down the velocity of the rise. A rise was never found to occur against the falling temperature, when in the neighbourhood of 50° F.

None of the above rules as to temperature were more strictly conformed to than that of the complete fall to winter level when the temperature passed below 50° F. In examining some hundreds of seasonal curves in about 20 of the largest towns of the three kingdoms, no exceptions, but one of a doubtful nature, were found to this rule, however early the rise of the epidemic occurred. The interesting and just perceptible tailing out of the epidemic frequently observed when the average weekly air temperature continued for several weeks at 50° F. or a little below, before falling decidedly, shows the tendency for some slight prevalence to continue as long as the temperature just remains above, or at, this point; *e.g.*, London and Sheffield, 1907; and London, Liverpool, Birmingham, and Glasgow, 1904. Above these limiting temperatures, however, with every degree of rise, there was found to be correspondingly greater potency in producing increase of prevalence.

(2) *Gradual Exhaustion of Epidemic Potential as the epidemic progresses: determining the typical explosive form of the mortality curve, and gradually reducing the degree of the reaction to temperature.*

The typically explosive form of the epidemic curve, very typical of an infectious disease (cf. also p. 113), has been carefully studied by Brownlee (1905–6) and others. It is, in effect, a graphic representation of the resultant between two opposing factors: firstly, the tendency to indefinitely continued multiplication of cases, which appears to proceed by regular geometrical progression (cf. Chart B, p. 120, Lond. 7 years); and secondly, an influence directly retarding this process, and acting throughout the epidemic so as to eventually bring about its complete cessation, at a rate, according to the authority named above, approaching to the terms of a geometrical progression. The question whether this retarding influence is dependent upon decrease in infective virulence of the causative organism or in the amount of susceptibility of the population, can be avoided by alluding to it as exhaustion of "epidemic potential," the latter term referring to the head of power for epidemic spread, present at any particular stage of the epidemic, as gauged by the highness of the infectivity over the lowness of the insusceptibility of the population. The resulting curve then, when not distorted by irregularities of temperature, has the well-known and characteristically regular form, with something of a rocket-like ascent, slowly and gracefully arching over to perhaps, though not necessarily, a rather more gradual fall (cf. Chart B, "The Explosive Curve").

The progressive exhaustion of epidemic potential introduces an influence qualifying, but be it noted in no sense disproving, the laws as to the effects of temperature above laid down. The movements of the curve are in fact completely dependent upon the precise inter-relation, at any given moment, of the two interacting factors: temperature, and degree of epidemic potential. It is obvious, from inspection of a typically explosive curve, that up to the moment the acme is reached, epidemic potential is a positive influence, producing increase in cases; after that point is passed, however, it is a negative one, producing a constant decrease. If then on the up-slope of the curve the temperature should be rising, an exaggerated effect upon the increase of prevalence would be produced, from the fact that the two separate influences are pulling together: whereas an exactly equal rise of temperature after the acme is passed would produce a much smaller effect, from the fact that the two influences are here in opposition. Conversely, a fall of temperature would produce the greatest visible effect upon the down-slope, and show the least result in diminution of cases upon the up-slope.

With this recognition of the two interacting factors, quite an interesting set of apparent anomalies of reactions to temperature are at once elucidated. Thus, the fact of a late diarrhoea epidemic forcing its way up for a few weeks after a moderate fall from summer temperatures has set in, will be seen, by applying the above principles, to be in no way incompatible with the constant controlling influence of temperature upon diarrhoea prevalence (cf. London, 1907 (Chart B), 1902, 1903, and 1905). Again, it is evident that if a rise to certain favourable summer temperatures should take place at the beginning of the season, and if these temperatures are thereafter maintained indefinitely at a constant level, the diarrhoea prevalence will not also be indefinitely maintained at a certain fixed level; but, as a matter of fact, the fixing of the temperature at a constant level merely serves to exclude the latter as a disturbing factor—exhaustion of epidemic potential being given full play to reveal itself in a perfect curve of typical explosive outline. Here, the influence of temperature, which becomes constant, would be of course responsible; firstly, for the fact that there should have been a rise at all; and secondly, for the highness of the point to which the epidemic curve rose, *i.e.*, for the highness of the acme. However, having been "drawn up," so to speak, to that highest possible point of prevalence, the curve would at once commence to descend in a regular manner, but always tending to indefinitely postpone the final and complete fall to winter level for as long as the air temperature maintained itself above the 50° F. limit. Thus besides rising against a falling temperature, the diarrhoea curve may also fall away from a maintained or even slightly rising temperature; both phenomena being still however consistent with a constant controlling temperature influence. Cf. London, 1898 (Chart B), 1899, 1895, and 1906, where these facts are most interestingly illustrated, and considerable falls in prevalence occur, during four or five weeks of high temperatures continuing at about 65° F., or even rising slowly to as high as 70° F.

Many of the London seasons were, however, so short as to give no opportunity of showing epidemic exhaustion; there can however be no doubt of its occurrence in such prolonged hot summers as those just mentioned. To establish however the matter altogether beyond question, a reference may be made to warmer countries having a much longer summer time, where a marked decline of the diarrhoea may commence as long as two months before the summer temperatures have reached their maximum (cf. Chart B, p. 120, Melb.). The most curious fact of the phenomenon is, that in different countries—in large cities at any rate—there is a tendency, probably depending to some extent upon a similar concentration of susceptible material in affected districts, for the time taken in the ascent to the maximum to be about the same in all cases, altogether without reference to the duration of the summer. Thus in the London charts the ascent averaged about seven weeks (cf. Chart B, Lond. 7 years and 1898); while in Melbourne it was again something under eight weeks (cf. Chart B, Melb.), although, owing to the longer summer, the epidemic in the latter instance lasted for 30 weeks, *i.e.*, twice as long as in London; the sudden uprush and rapid falling away from the acme, as if the epidemic had over-reached itself, is thus very marked; this being followed by a more leisurely fall, although the temperature is still rising for two months or more, and the winter level is not reached till 50° F. has been passed, just as in London.

Again, from the fact that the greatest velocity of the curve is found on the two slopes just below the summit; and the least, at the summit and towards the base; notchings due to sudden alterations in temperature are graphically most apparent in the latter positions; very great alterations of temperature being required to produce notchings upon the slopes. The frequently observed sudden falling away, when the acme is passed, is also explained by the above fact of the very great velocity of the curve at that particular point, and also by the fact that, in the data presented, there was generally a falling temperature at that time helping to accelerate the descent.

Finally, it also follows, that the greatness of the height to which the curve rises, *i.e.*, of the maximum weekly prevalence attained, is proportionate, other things being equal, to the general height of the temperature plateau from which it rises. Thus, the tallest curve in a series of seasons, if other factors were not unequal, should be the one where there was not only a very high temperature during the week of maximum prevalence, but where also there had been generally high temperatures for some time preceding, leading up—uninterruptedly— to the week of the acme. Cf. 1904 and 1897, London, which bear this out. From these and other considerations it is apparent why comparisons between epidemic prevalence and the average temperature of the third quarter do not give very regular results: additional information as to the highest temperature attained would help the comparison. Again, in cold seasons, where the epidemic is abnormally late in appearance, it practically always happens that the rise when it occurs is from a comparatively low plateau of temperature. Hence the almost invariable absence of tallness in these curves. While from the fact that the fall to 50° F. seldom takes place much later than in other seasons, it happens that they are also short in length, *i.e.*, in duration (cf. Chart B, London, 1907). Such epidemics, rising from low temperature levels, are therefore almost invariably of insignificant proportions. Yet, from the deferred date of onset, it might be contended that the susceptibility of the population, and the consequent degree of epidemic potential, would be even greater than in the warm early season, so that the epidemic might be expected to exhibit great expansive power and to continue to exist beyond the temperature limits observed in other seasons. The fact that it certainly does not do this provides therefore a demonstration, in another way, that *the explosive power* of an epidemic, *as well as the amount of prevalence*, depends for its existence upon, and *varies directly with, the height of the accompanying temperature*.

Brownlee (1905–6), in testing the fit of epidemic curves to various theoretical distributions, found that in composite curves of diarrhoea for long series of years in London and Glasgow, a good fit could not be obtained at the apices. This is evidently due to the disturbing influence of changes of temperature upon the normal evolution of the explosive curve. Thus, the temperature during the ascent of the curve, is generally rising; the rate of rise is therefore being continually increased, and the apex of the curve is drawn up higher, with a steeper up-slope, than it would otherwise have been had the temperature remained constant. Again, since the apices of the composite temperature and diarrhoea curves will probably not coincide (cf. Chart B, p. 120, Lond. seven years' curve)—the temperature tending to fall a little earlier or later than the diarrhoea—the apex of the latter curve will be accordingly asymmetrical, being pulled over to one side or the other.

(3) *The suggested inter-relation of Temperature, Flies, and Diarrhoea.*

Of the all-importance of temperature in this epidemic disease there can be no kind of doubt; and it was well to follow out its relations to diarrhoea prevalence to complete finality before introducing the discussion of fly-carriage and other indirect means through which it is suggested the effects of temperature are produced.

The suggested influence of fly-carriage must now be considered at some length, so as to determine what part of, or whether the whole of, the phenomena of the epidemic and mortality sickness curves, above noted, might be referable to and can be completely explained by this factor, including of course both the varying effects of temperature, and the phenomena of epidemic exhaustion. Curves of fly prevalence are now available for comparison with the diarrhoea mortality curve for five years at Manchester (Niven: 1904–6, 1908–9), and three years at London

(Hamer: 1908–10); and it will be interesting, and somewhat necessary, to compare the above observed relations of temperature and diarrhoea with a possible third relation to fly prevalence, from the evidence collected by these observers. There is on casual inspection a general correspondence in the general form, and in the notchings, of the fly and diarrhoea curves for any one year; but this might be attributed simply to both being dependent upon a common influence, the temperature, without there being necessarily any real causal relationship between them themselves. If the seasonal prevalence of flies determines *all* the phenomena of the epidemic curve, then by far the most reasonable conclusion to be deduced from this would be that the diarrhoea curve should be found to follow *exactly* the outline of the fly curve. *This it does not do in any* of the eight separate seasons above mentioned. The diarrhoea curve varies from the fly curve chiefly in two respects,—

(1)   Firstly, *the response of the diarrhoea curve to the rise of the fly curve is a very tardy one,* and *the rate of rise is different.* Some slight rise is generally evident about the time of the earliest increase in fly prevalence; but in three of the seasons (London 1908, 1909, and Manchester 1906) periods of three weeks elapsed before any considerable response of the diarrhoea curve was visible, or five weeks before the main rise in deaths took place (cf. Chart B, p. 120, Lond. 1908–9). Several of the records do not show the early and late relations of the two curves. This lagging behind the rise of fly prevalence is very similar then to the lagging of the diarrhoea behind the temperature, on its first rise to summer level, as discussed in a preceding section (p. 122 *et seq.*). For explanation of this occurrence there seems to be no need to go further than suppose that, whatever the means by which the high degree of temperature, or the fly prevalence, "draws up" the curve, the utmost degree of prevalence they have power to induce cannot be induced forthwith, but has to be patiently evolved by multiplication from an amount of infection of relatively microscopic proportions; this multiplication being in the nature of a geometrical progression, as suggested by the usual rate of increase as the main rise becomes definitely established (cf. Chart B, Lond. 7 yrs.). When once however the terms of this progression have reached an appreciable size, the charted curve shows that apparently sudden upward rush so characteristic of a graphic representation of this mode of multiplication, and the rate of increase of diarrhoea soon outstrips the rate of increase of flies: for the increase of flies more closely approaches an ordinary arithmetical progression, each of the slopes of the fly curve tending, to some extent, to approximate to a

straight line (cf. Chart B, Lond. Composite curves, 1908–9). Since however the temperature is not generally constant during the ascent of the fly curve, but is usually rising a little, it follows that there may be irregular acceleration of this arithmetical rate of increase, with consequent curving inwards of the upward slope. The lagging behind of the diarrhoea, and subsequent outstripping of the fly increase, produces a curving or sagging inward of the diarrhoea up-slope, away from the up-slope of the fly curve; an appearance which is actually observed or suggested in *every one* of the eight seasonal records provided (cf. Chart. B), and there can therefore be no doubt as to the reality of its occurrence.

In accepting the above view of the matter, we are furnished with a second and most important demonstration (cf. Sect. V, 4, p. 65) of the fact that the infection of the disease does not arrive on the bodies of the flies from the manure or refuse heaps in which they are bred: in which case the up-slope of the diarrhoea curve would follow quite closely the course of the fly curve: on the contrary, the rise of the diarrhoea curve, by geometrical progression, almost certainly relates to the origin and multiplication of infection by transmission from person to person.

(2) Secondly, *the rate of fall of the diarrhoea curve is also different*, the down-slope sagging inwards away from the fly curve, as happened also on the up-slope. There can be no doubt again as to the occurrence of this difference; it is also observed, or suggested, *in every one* of the eight records (cf. Chart. B, London curves, 1908 and 1909); and thus it is evident that the phenomenon of epidemic exhaustion, in part at least, could not be explained by exhaustion of the function of multiplication of flies in protracted summers, or by any cause, such as disease of the flies themselves, which might produce the fall in fly prevalence. At the period of maximum prevalence the dissemination of infective matter throughout the population, is also at its maximum; the diarrhoea, therefore, if there were no such deterrent as exhaustion of susceptible persons or of the infectivity of the causative organism, should thereafter necessarily follow closely, if not actually pass above, the outline of the fly curve; and only decrease when forced down by, and in close company with, the decline of fly prevalence. The fact that, after passing the acme, it fell away from the fly curve, necessarily proves the presence of some unexplained factor, apart from fly prevalence; and this rapid falling away from the acme, so characteristic of the decline of the typical explosive curve, before alluded to, at once points to intrinsic exhaustion of epidemic

potential as the factor in question[1]. In addition, however, there is quite possibly some exhaustion or falling away of the fly prevalence from the temperature in protracted hot summers; as it is difficult not to believe that the function of fly multiplication has also natural limitations to its seasonal rage, notwithstanding the maintenance of favourable summer temperatures: as in the case of exhaustion of florification of early flowering plants. There is a slight suggestion of this in one season only. Data collected in warm countries having longer summers where epidemic exhaustion is exhibited weeks and months before the mid-summer temperature is reached should give interesting information on this point; or even London data, if fly counts could be made in such a protracted summer as 1899. The undoubted existence of intrinsic exhaustion in diarrhoea makes it plain that indefinitely continued multiplication of flies will not be accompanied by a similar indefinite increase in diarrhoea cases: at the lower levels of prevalence there is possibly, however, a fairly definite relation between the numbers of flies and the numbers of cases.

The continued rise of diarrhoea after the decline of summer temperatures has set in has been noted as a phenomenon of the epidemic curve not inconsistent with a strong controlling influence of temperature. A similar continued rise against temperature for two or three weeks is observable in the fly curve, closely accompanying and afterwards declining with the diarrhoea curve, in 1907 and 1908 at London, and in 1905 and 1908 at Manchester. As in the case of diarrhoea, the strong controlling influence of temperature is invariably evidenced in a rapid decrease in the rate of multiplication; but in the above examples, from the fact that the temperature did not fall to sufficiently unfavourable levels, the decrease in the rate was not ocularly demonstrated upon the chart as an actual fall of the curve, as it was not sufficient to produce at once a smaller number of flies in the weeks immediately following the fall of temperature.

This occurrence has important bearing upon the question as to whether other factors, including the degree of *activity of flies*, upon which temperature may have some effect, are as important as the relative number of flies present. The writer (1908, p. 37) was led to suggest the probable importance of the former factor from noticing the

---

[1] The falling away of the diarrhoea curve, and the possible explanation of exhaustion of susceptible persons, has been mentioned by Niven (1910). The fact was noted here, however, and Chart B, Lond. 1908–9, was constructed, before acquaintance was made with that paper. See reference at foot of this paper.

marked precipitation of flies upon doors and window-frames upon sudden falls of temperature to somewhere below 54° F.; a phenomenon which, further, may afford a reasonable explanation of the curious fact of the almost immediate drop in the numbers of flies caught and of cases of diarrhoea occurring with a fall of temperature. In the above examples of seasons, however, the fall of temperature must have decreased the activity of flies; the fact that the increase of diarrhoea, notwithstanding, continued as long as the increase in flies also continued, showed that the diarrhoea varied with the numbers of flies rather than with the amount of movement of the flies—the latter factor thus apparently being, at most, one of only subordinate importance : all this of course being subject to ultimate proof of the fly carrier theory. It might again be suggested that, in approaching the acme, the higher rate of increase of diarrhoea than of fly prevalence is due to the increased activity of flies at the higher temperatures which generally prevail about that time, increasing thereby the infective potentialities of the flies. But this objection cannot be seriously entertained : for, apart from any slight bearing upon the matter of the observation as to the rise against temperature made above, it is also obvious from most of the prevalence data that a definite difference exists in the rate of rise of the two curves, whatever be the movement of the temperature. Thus, in Chart B, Lond. 1908–9, during the three weeks preceding the week of maximum diarrhoea prevalence—which were those in which the whole of the outstripping of the fly curve took place—there was actually a slightly falling temperature.

All the foregoing, as to the inter-relations of diarrhoea, fly prevalence, and temperature, is essentially contained in the following three facts (cf. Chart B, Lond. 1908–9):

(1) *All three curves are definitely correlated one to the other; but the fly curve is more closely correlated to the temperature curve than the diarrhoea curve is*, getting more rapidly into relation with it at the early part of the season and appearing more loath to fall away from it later on; its behaviour being apparently quite compatible with the theory that fly prevalence is an intermediary factor between temperature and diarrhoea.

(2) *The fly curve, however, does not render an absolutely mechanical obedience to its controlling influence—the temperature, but shows great independence of movement*, dependent upon intrinsic factors, concerned, amongst other things, with the exigencies of fly breeding. Thus, it both lags behind the temperature in rising, owing to the time taken in the

multiplying process; and shows small response to rises of temperature on the falling curve, from the fly prevalence being largely subject to the egg-laying of several weeks before. Both these features were also present in diarrhoea, but in a somewhat magnified degree for reasons next to be discussed.

(3) *In the same way*, it is important to note, *the diarrhoea curve also shows some independence of movement of*—what may prove to be its controlling factor—*the fly prevalence*, owing to the intrusion of certain intrinsic factors: lagging behind the rising fly curve, from the inertia of case-to-case multiplication; and falling away from it later on from exhaustion of infection or of the material to infect.

An explanation is afforded by the latter facts, and by others formerly given, why, if the number of flies becomes stationary on the ascending curve, the diarrhoea may continue to rise; while, if occurring on the descending slope, the diarrhoea curve may continue to fall, sometimes also appearing to fall away before the acme of fly prevalence is reached. A similar relation of diarrhoea has already been noted with regard to a stationary temperature (cf. p. 125). Again, just as with regard to temperature, if we could eliminate variations of fly prevalence by imagining a high fly prevalence evenly maintained throughout the season, the diarrhoea curve would be seen to rush up to it, and then fall away, with the typically explosive outline.

Finally, it is important to note that the diarrhoea curve—although at first falling more quickly than the fly curve—later on, however, tails out, so as not to finally collapse till about the same time as the fly curve; that is, about the time the weekly air temperature passes decidedly below 50° F. Only two of the records are however continued long enough to give any indication as to whether at this point the level of fly prevalence becomes low enough to be disregarded as a factor exerting any positive influence.

A striking fact which specially deserves to be mentioned in connection with fly-carriage of diarrhoea was noted by the writer in examining charts of the great cholera epidemics of London in 1849, 1854, and 1866. They appeared to be governed by exactly the same temperature conditions as diarrhoea and to vary in the same way with variations of temperature. Particularly noticeable was the quite simultaneous subsidence of the two diseases as 50° F. was passed. Similar temperature effects upon multiplication of the respective organisms in food or water might of course be urged in explanation. But in view of the widely differing temperature limitations of cholera in various other countries the above facts are highly suggestive—even allowing for some confusion in diagnosis of the two diseases—of the common influence of fly-carriage in both.

Another fact, with regard to the pre-epidemic period, appears to fit in well with the fly hypothesis. It will be recalled that at air temperatures of 60° F. or a little below (cf. p. 119), the first two weeks of this period pass without any sign of increase of cases of diarrhoea, or a longer period at lower temperatures; afterwards a slight increase leads up to the main rise. Fly-counts, such as at London, 1909 and 1908, and at Manchester, 1906 and 1904, also indicate a corresponding interval or its equivalent before increase of flies occurs: and 14 days, at such temperatures, is just about the period necessary from the laying of eggs to the hatching of the first brood of flies. Thus Newstead (1907, p. 16) says: "The whole cycle from egg to perfect insect occupies, under the most favourable conditions, from 10 to 14 days; but in low temperatures the whole cycle may extend to several weeks."

In conclusion it might be stated that of the various points of non-correspondence of the fly and diarrhoea curves noted here, none of them have been found impossible of explanation, so as to be incompatible with a theory of fly-carriage; although causation is not necessarily thereby established. The same applies to the objections noted in a former paper (1908), which, with the help of the four additional sets of data since provided, particularly those of London for 1908 and 1909, mostly appear to be at least capable of explanation on the principles above laid down. An ambiguous sentence (*ibid.* pp. 36, 37) contained in the above, which was marked for revision but finally escaped notice, as to the balance of epidemiological evidence being unfavourable to the fly theory, referred, as the accompanying context suggests, to the evidence of the fly curves then available, and not to the large amount of epidemiological evidence of other kinds. The concluding sentence, which may just as aptly be applied to the conclusion of the present section, refers to the correspondences of temperature, flies and diarrhoea, as being so extraordinary "that the whole question merits the most thorough and laborious investigation" (*ibid.* p. 37).

The suggested correspondence, both in rise and decline, of the 4-ft. Earth Temperature tracing with the Diarrhoea Curve.

It might be well to again insist on the fact that any correspondence of the 4-ft. earth temperature tracing with the curve of diarrhoea prevalence, *e.g.*, as regards the very frequent attainment in this country of their maxima at the same time, and any correspondence in commencement of fall (cf. Ballard, 1887—8, p. 3), are quite unessential facts as regards causation ; as they wholly depend upon the mere chance agreement, in the short summers of this country, of the length of the interval occupied in rising to the acme of the temperature curve, with the length of the interval by the end of which the diarrhoea epidemic has usually ascended to its acme, and begins to show signs of exhaustion by descent of the curve (cf. 7 yrs. Lond. in Chart B, p. 120). In countries having protracted summers—judging their length by the amount of time passed above a certain temperature level—the diarrhoea may reach its maximum, and begin to decline, more than two months before the 4-ft. temperature has reached its maximum (Armstrong, 1905, p. 517).

Again, with regard to the rise of diarrhoea and its relation to the 4-ft. earth temperature, objection must also be taken to the assertion, without proper qualification, that the 4-ft. temperature furnishes a register of cumulative temperature. That may be apparent in a few seasons where an interrupted rise of temperature has taken place, and is still taking place, but where, through remissions of temperature, the 4-ft. record has once become stationary during its ascent, or has fallen, all account is lost of the amount of heat received during that check, and such irregularities occur in the majority of the short and irregular seasons of this country. The 56° F. standard certainly furnishes a sign very easily determined and very intelligible to the inexpert, in comparison with the accumulated air temperature standard, which is somewhat difficult to estimate, and to express in brief concise terms. But notwithstanding, in the former case, so many exceptions have to be explained away, and so many adjustments to be made, that it is doubtful if it possesses much advantage in these respects over the latter, even apart from its very questionable adaptation as a scientific test (cf. also p. 686, and Chart B, Lond., 1907). In records and charts of diarrhoea prevalence, where one temperature record only can be included, it should unquestionably be that of the *air* temperature. Such a preference is the one most consistent with a strictly scientific view of the matter ; since the air temperature is the one most directly connected with diarrhoea prevalence, and also shows the best correspondence to the fluctuations and fall of the diarrhoea curve (due allowance having been made for the explosive contour of the latter). Both the 4-ft. and 1-ft. earth temperatures may, however, be also usefully included.

The suggested influence of the 4-ft. Earth Temperature, upon Diarrhoea Prevalence, through its suggested direct relation to Fly Prevalence.

Similar care is needed, to that enjoined above, in interpreting apparent correspondences between the fly curve and the 4-ft. temperature tracing; and any attempt to explain the apparent inter-relation of the diarrhoea and 4-ft. temperature curves, by bringing into prominence a direct effect of the 4-ft. earth temperature upon fly-breeding, without clear and sufficient warrant for doing so, tends only to re-introduce confusion into these matters.

It is difficult to understand how the latter temperature can have much influence upon the dates of *commencement* and *completion* of seasonal fly prevalence, even in the districts where there are many privies and manure-pits sunk in the ground. Firstly, the deep earth temperature is notably lower than superficial earth temperature at the beginning of summer; therefore, the first swarms of flies will not come from such situations but rather from heated manure lying more superficially; and secondly, though at the close of the season with the earth temperatures comparatively higher than the air temperatures, sunken pits would enable the development of fly larvae to continue, yet, seeing that fly pupae are generally deposited near the surface, the influence of such pits will be largely neutralized by the fact that the emergence of fresh swarms of flies will be completely subject to, and inhibited by, the comparatively low air temperature.

The primary fact of the seasonal rise and decline of fly prevalence appears to be the direct effect of the *air temperature* upon the imago or adult insect, determining its first emergence, and its final immobilization; and to a less extent upon the pupae: both of these are habitually more or less exposed to its influence. Otherwise, as regards the larvae and eggs, there is as much hot manure in winter as in summer for developing the larvae, but the lowness of the temperature in winter immobilises the adult fly, and so prevents the laying of eggs.

The almost immediate response of the numbers of flies to the fall and rise of temperature is very curious: if not wholly due to the effect of variations of temperature upon the amount of fly movement, it may possibly be due to some extent to the flies going into their hiding places, as they are supposed to do in the winter time, upon the supervention of a cold change—especially if of a gradual kind, and emerging at once on a change to warmer weather. Otherwise, the prevalence of any one week appears to depend upon two factors: firstly, upon the favourableness of the temperature for egg-laying two, three, or more weeks before; and secondly, upon the favourableness of the present temperature for emergence from the pupae. It so happens, therefore, that past and present temperatures may sometimes counteract each other with regard to their effect upon prevalence.

The influence of rainfall upon diarrhoea prevalence need not be discussed further than to say that its influence is probably almost wholly produced by its effect in reducing the temperature: this should, of course, react secondarily upon diarrhoea prevalence. From a few obervations the writer has made it appears that its influence in driving flies indoors depends wholly upon whether during the fall of rain the temperature indoors is warmer than without; if cooler, the flies appear to remain outside. On comparing the meteorological and prevalence charts for Mansfield, there certainly does appear to be some amount of correspondence with rainfall. It is not certain however that irregular periods of collection of the data had not a good deal to do with this (cf. also paper, 1908, pp. 12, 13).

(ii)   *Influences determining the outline of the Diarrhoea Sickness Curve.*

The preceding remarks upon the mortality curve appear to apply equally as regards the effect of temperature and the exhaustion of epidemic potential, to the curve of prevalence of *all cases* of diarrhoea; the latter yielding confirmatory evidence upon these points.

A comparison of *Ballard's* (1887–8) *returns of diarrhoea sickness* for 10 years (1857–66) at Islington, with Greenwich air temperatures, bears out the conclusions on these points: epidemic explosiveness and exhaustion are particularly well illustrated. The years 1858, 1862, and 1866, show the epidemic continuing to rise for one and two four-weekly periods after the maximum temperature has been passed. In one year, 1865 the epidemic prevalence fell rapidly, while the temperature was maintained or still rose slightly, for two more of such periods. Moreover, 50° F. appeared to be the limiting temperature. The two most insignificant outbreaks, 1860 and 1862, were those in which the highest average temperature reached only 58° F. and 60° F. respectively, and for one monthly period in each. The tallest curve, 1859 (excluding the cholera year 1866), surmounted the highest four-weekly temperatures of the whole series. There were no notchings of the curves except in one instance, owing no doubt to the length of the periods taken, so that the effects of small variations of temperature were thus not observable, although the effects of larger variations were to be seen in the ways above noted, as also in the steepness of slopes of different curves.

The *Mansfield data* will now be similarly examined.

(1) *Irregular evolution in point of time of the epidemic, in different districts and neighbourhoods.*

Although, a short time after the arrival of the air temperature at 60° F., simultaneous appearance or increase of cases occurred generally throughout the town, *i.e.*, in 13 out of 15 localities visited (cf. p. 111), these cases were nevertheless comparatively few and scattered, and the main seasonal outbursts in the various districts did not follow, in some instances, until considerable periods had elapsed; the outbursts in different districts, again, occurring at widely different dates, and the dates of attainment of the maximum prevalence also differing to a certain extent. Similar differences are apparent between the subdivisions of a large city, when compared as regards mortality, as illustrated in the writer's former paper (1908, Chart VIII), the differences being less, the larger the divisions taken: hence the greater reliability of massive statistics (cf. also pp. 46 and 95).

Such differences may be explained in one or more of the following ways: firstly, they may depend upon the transference between different districts of specially virulent strains of infection. The main outbursts may be so determined, while the scattered low prevalence found on all sides during the season may be due to widespread strains of only ordinary virulence. Secondly, they may depend more upon such strains of infection gaining access at varying dates to centres of highly susceptible people. Thirdly, they may depend wholly upon irregular local prevalences of flies.

It may be briefly stated that from careful observations upon this matter a general conviction was received as to the frequent applicability of the first, and to some extent of the second; but irregular local development of fly prevalence did not appear to be an important factor, although it is quite possible that it may have frequently played such a part (cf. also p. 67).

Some details as to irregular evolution in the several districts may now be given.

The main rise in the quadrilateral did not occur till more than four weeks later than in the triangle—and this was distinctly not due to later visitation and collection of data in that area, appearing also to continue till a correspondingly later period; a certain number of scattered cases had however occurred from as early a date as in the latter district. As regards other parts of the town, the main rises were found to occur at widely different times; but most of them, it may be noted, occurred more about the same time as that of the quadrilateral than at any other. Area III (Charts III and IV, App.) began a week later, and Area IV (Chart IV, App.) a week earlier.

Although there was good reason to believe that in several other foci there were also a large number of cases occurring as early in the season as the main rise in the triangle, yet the great contrast in date of onset, between the comparatively large and important outbreaks in the triangle and in the quadrilateral is a very remarkable fact. Differences in temperature, owing to altitude, are not marked enough to account for it: Area IV with a three weeks later epidemic being not so elevated as the triangle: and at the same time it is evident that the rule as to a fixed period of cumulative temperatures is widely diverged from in the case of the ultimate local units or foci of the epidemic wave; pointing away from a general and mechanically precise reaction of ground organisms to temperature, to case-to-case methods of spread, and also to irregular transplantation of strains of infection of varying virulence.

It is interesting to note that the groundwork of the charts between the specially virulent foci is filled up by a large number of scattered cases, which from their isolated nature, in spite of apparent susceptible material close at hand, are presumably of very low infective virulence.

The analysis of the outbreak in each of the two large districts shows great divergences in date of outburst in different neighbourhoods, and suggests even a possible perambulation of infection from one part to another. When the quadrilateral is divided into five districts to best set off these occurrences, the outburst is seen to be curiously later and later in each neighbourhood, on going north; as if spread had occurred in that direction from the few virulent outbreaks—one of which was imported as previously described—that had occurred in the first section at a comparatively early date in the season. Again, in the triangle where the distribution of the epidemic naturally occurred in three divisions (Chart V, App.), the second division appeared to derive its infection from the first by gradual passage from the very early outbreak in a Street, along β Street, to δ Street. These may only be coincidences, but still, occurring as they do in both districts, they are worth calling attention to.

(2) *Effect of Temperature in producing variations in prevalence of Diarrhoea Sickness.*

The sickness data of a town of considerable size would of course require to be furnished in order to consistently demonstrate the influence of temperature, which as has been before suggested is of a very general kind; its effects in producing variations in prevalence, when only small districts are taken, being frequently smothered by the irregular firing off of the various component foci of infection. In the data here presented, many of the dates of attack were only approximate, the attacks being referred to indefinitely as having occurred in the middle, or at the end of, a certain week : such cases were respectively placed under Wednesdays or Thursdays, and Sundays; which gives an excessive incidence upon these days. However, many general variations corresponding with temperature can be found upon a not over-critical study of the charts. Thus, the cessation of epidemic prevalence can be made out about the time the air temperature passed decidedly below 50° F. Again, the most marked variation in temperature during the season was the very unseasonable rise at the end of September, following after a period of rather low and intermittent temperatures. In correspondence with this the curve of diarrhoea for both districts shows a late rise. The curve for the triangle, again, is mainly composed of three humps corresponding with three similar elevations of temperature (particularly as regards maximum temperatures) during the period of highest temperatures, from about June 22 to August 9. After the latter date there was a fall, followed by a slight rise in both temperature and cases, particularly between August 16 and 30; and then a sudden fall of cases almost to zero, accompanying a fall in temperature to somewhere about the limiting temperature of 50° F.

(3) *Evidence of Epidemic Exhaustion.*

The foregoing remarks as to the great divergence in dates of outburst in different neighbourhoods and districts may now be completed by the addition of the important observation that almost as a general rule *early local outbreaks were correspondingly early in coming to an end* or in falling to a low prevalence, in spite of the continued maintenance of favourable temperatures; and late outbreaks were correspondingly late. The conclusion suggested is that in the former case the epidemic has worked itself out early, by exhaustion of susceptible persons, or of infective virulence in the causal organism; for there is not infrequently marked absence of cases in such neighbourhoods for the rest of the season, as well as before. In fact the entire epidemic in the two districts appears to be almost wholly made up of a number of these small local explosions, isolated in point of time as well as of place and each about three weeks in length.

This exhaustion in small foci is evidently then the expression in miniature, and the foundation of, the similar phenomenon exhibited in the curve of total prevalence for a large district, or for a whole city: this matter, which has already been fully demonstrated with regard to the mortality data, will also be found to lend itself readily to demonstration from the point of view of sickness data.

All the above facts are very clearly exhibited in Charts IV, V, and VII, App.; the local outbreaks referred to are as a matter of fact the place and time groups discussed on p. 88 *et seq.* The two main facts to be noted are; firstly, in Chart VII, it is seen that however early the outbreak in one of these clumps was placed in the season, the clump as a whole was practically never attacked again during the rest of the year, and even solitary cases were very infrequent; secondly, notwithstanding the wholesale prevalence on every hand, 86% of the cases were not attacked a second time during the season, and 96% had no second attack more than six weeks after the first. From these two points *a conclusion as to the reality of epidemic exhaustion by exhaustion of susceptible persons is unavoidable.* It is evident that generally speaking the epidemic cannot, or at least does not, attack where it has been before in the same season. If then the infective virulence remains constant, it necessarily follows that as the season progresses the number of susceptibles diminishes, the distance between them increases, and the chance of attack consequently becomes continually smaller.

Comparing now the individual prevalences of the two large districts, it is at once seen that *the outbreak in the triangle is a remarkable illustration, on an extensive scale, of early exhaustion of the diarrhoea epidemic.* In both districts the main epidemic was limited to about the same period, *i.e.*, eight weeks; but the one in the triangle, commencing four weeks earlier than that in the quadrilateral, was exhausted—at least to a very low prevalence—four weeks earlier, notwithstanding the fact that both districts evidently shared the same temperature conditions. Again, it will be seen that even the quadrilateral, which had an epidemic as late as that in most parts of the town, showed weakened response to rises of temperature as the epidemic progressed; the outbreak in the southern half being finished particularly early. And indeed the argument from small foci to large districts, and from large districts to the whole town, naturally follows without the necessity of further demonstration; particularly as it has been shown that the disease was already scattered through every part of the town from the very commencement of the season.

Moreover, all the other peculiar effects due to the interaction of temperature and the typical explosive epidemic, which were noticed in regard to the mortality curve, are also individually evident with regard to these sickness data. Thus, some local explosions, which happened to commence just as a fall to low temperatures had taken place, continued to rise notwithstanding. Cf. the explosion in the week ending August 22, on the curve of the triangle, which was wholly confined to one neighbourhood. Again, the curve, even with these limited data, is seen to be decidedly *rounded off*, in descent as well as in ascent, not exhibiting, moreover, mechanical and sharply cut reactions to temperature variations. *The tendency to a typical explosive curve*, exhibiting epidemic exhaustion and all its other characteristic features, *is thus unmistakably revealed.*

As regards explanations of epidemic exhaustion, other than that of exhaustion of susceptible persons, *exhaustion of infective virulence of the causative organisms* might be suggested; but in this case it might have been expected that neighbourhoods in which an outbreak had worked itself out would frequently have been re-attacked later in the season, from the spread from adjacent or distant neighbourhoods of new and fully virulent strains of infection. But second outbreaks in these clumps were exceedingly uncommon. The manifesting of exhaustion after the end of eight weeks from the rise, a period of similar length being found in different countries in spite of long-continued high temperatures in some, is however of peculiar interest with respect to the above matter (cf. p. 125). Again, the question of small local decreases in fly prevalence need not be considered, from the fact that clumps, attacked at widely different dates, were frequently closely adjacent. Moreover, as regards the four weeks earlier exhaustion in the triangle than in the quadrilateral, it is difficult to believe that the fly swarms were exhausted or were willing to leave so attractive a district as the triangle thus early in the season, or that if they were, that swarms from neighbouring districts would not have freely migrated into it to fill their places. *Exhaustion of epidemic potential apart from decrease in flies*, which was demonstrated without doubt with regard to the relations of the mortality and fly curves (cf. p. 127 *et seq.*) is thus demonstrated with almost equal certainty from the sickness data.

Finally, it might be noted that the definite amount of acquired immunity found in Sect. III, 5 to follow attack, along with the above facts, suggests that exhaustion of susceptible persons was by far the most important factor in the question. Some explanation is, however, required of the bald statement given above, that the early collapse in the triangle or in the southern part of the quadrilateral was due to exhaustion of susceptible persons. It is not for a moment suggested that there were not numbers of persons left unattacked who would have succumbed to the disease had fair opportunity been given. That is evident from its behaviour in π Street, where, after a moderate prevalence similar to that in other parts of the district, the disease, so to speak, broke out again, 25 out of 58 persons in houses 4—16, *i.e.*, nearly half, being attacked. A similarly severe incidence was also found there in 1909. A high incidence, similar to that found in 1908, was also found in γ Street in 1909. It appears then that, in certain dirty parts of the town, almost everyone might be attacked once in two or three years. On the other hand, there is reason to believe that in clean parts many people may go on from year to year without having the disease at all, and yet they must necessarily possess less acquired immunity than the people who are so frequently subject to attack. It is evident then that, as suggested before, *the question of exhaustion of susceptibility of a population is altogether a relative matter.* It does not depend wholly upon individual immunity, and upon the virulence of the infection, but upon the *total resistance* offered by these and *various other factors*. Thus, in a clean area, the resistance to spread is so great, that whatever infection enters, dies, so to speak, an early death; being able to reach only those who present an extraordinarily high degree of susceptibility; and probably even missing the greater part of these, from want of ready means of dissemination. In a dirty district, however, free course is given to the infection. Nevertheless, as evidenced also in the dirtiest parts of the triangle, there is a limit here also, and the outbreak will generally fail and disappear for the rest of the season before half of the people are attacked.

Epidemic exhaustion is particularly well shown in the early and heavily attacked a and β Streets (Nos. 1—35 and Nos. 41—63). Only one case occurred, in the season, after August 19, while in the quadrilateral nearly half the attacks, and in the whole town nearly all the diarrhoea deaths, occurred after this date. In *a* Street, where the houses were very dirty, and where the earliest explosive outburst occurred, 14 persons had been attacked in the ten houses, and the epidemic was practically over for the rest of the season by July 15, before the hottest of the summer, which preceded the outburst in the quadrilateral and in District III, had arrived. Further, the question of immunity might be expected to have some bearing upon determining the distribution of attacked houses into clumps, and also to qualify the results of many of the analytical tables throughout this paper. There has not been time to completely follow out all these matters; but from a cursory examination, it appears that no material qualification of any of the conclusions arrived at would be caused thereby.

(c) *Conclusions as to factors governing Epidemic Prevalence.*

(1) *The " Ground" theory versus the " Fly-Carrier" theory.*

As regards the various interpretations, above given, of the phenomena both of epidemic rise and decline, an attempt will now be made to decide *which combination* of such interpretations *most closely coincides with the facts at present available.* The matter is rendered somewhat complex by the introduction of the opposing theories of ground infection and personal infection; and the various possible interpretations have, for the sake of clearness, been tabulated below.

A.—The temperature phenomena of the two periods may be interpreted in one or more of several different ways, as follow:

The pre-epidemic period:

(i) As being occupied in maturing a high degree of infectivity in a ground organism.

(ii) As necessary to the production of effective swarms of fly carriers.

The epidemic period: the temperature notchings and limitations may be interpreted—

(iii) As a direct effect upon the infective virulence of the crop of ground organisms from which all epidemic cases might prove to be directly derived.

(iv) As a direct effect upon the infective virulence of the organism, during the brief interval of exposure, in passage from person to person.

(v) As a direct effect upon the prevalence of fly-carriers.

B.—Epidemic Exhaustion may be interpreted in one or more of the following ways:

(i) As exhaustion of infective virulence of a ground organism, as it lies in or on the ground: infectivity being a function with seasonal limitations, like as in the flowering of plants.

(ii) As exhaustion of infective virulence in an organism, personally transmitted.

(iii) As exhaustion of susceptible persons; whether the organism be derived from a ground or from a personal source.

Before proceeding to discuss the relative values of the above hypotheses a brief recapitulation will be made of the few facts of the disease, the certainty of which the evidence of this or of other enquiries might claim to have unquestionably established.

A Statement of Known Facts.

(1) There *is* a constantly controlling and facultatively inhibitive force, exercised by temperature (cf. pp. 119, 139, etc.).

(2) There *is* exhaustion of epidemic potential, apart from the decline of fly prevalence (cf. p. 127 *et seq.*).

(3) There *is* undoubtedly a good deal of acquired immunity in the population; and this will account for some part of the phenomenon of epidemic decline (cf. p. 139 *et seq.*).

(4) There *is* undoubtedly a good deal of transmission of infection from person to person (see p. 115, Summary).

(5) There *is* widespread infection to be found from the very beginning of the season, that is, at least from the end of the pre epidemic period (cf. p. 111).

(6) There *is* also a definite pre-epidemic period of favourable temperatures, during which diarrhoea appears to undergo practically no increase—at least, at all comparable to the rate found at the time of the main rise (cf. p. 119).

To these facts of positive import may be added a few of a negative character:

(7) We have *no* knowledge, at present, of such occurrences as that of a direct effect of temperature upon infectivity during transmission from case to case (see *A* (iv) above).

(8) There are, at present, few facts to support a theory as to exhaustion of infectivity, during repeated passage of organisms from person to person throughout the season (see *B* (ii) above).

(9) No evidence was found in this paper adverse to the fly-carrier theory. On the other hand a great deal of indirect evidence was obtained in its' favour. The extent of correlation of the prevalence curves of flies and diarrhoea appeared to be quite compatible with the fly theory (cf. p. 127 *et seq.*).

In view of the first two negative considerations just mentioned, two of the possible explanations on p. 143 *et seq.*, viz.:—*A* (iv) and *B* (ii), may, at present, be practically excluded: and *with the exclusion of theory A* (iv) *the possibility of direct personal infection explaining the whole phenomenon of prevalence is also excluded.*

The question is thereby rendered much less complex, and *the choice is practically left between two principal combinations*, which are as follow :

(1) A combination of explanations *A* (i), *A* (iii), and *B* (i); which is, in effect, the *" ground "* theory.

(2) A combination of the remaining explanations *A* (ii), *A* (v), and *B* (iii), which is, in effect, the *" fly-carrier "* theory. Several other combinations of the theories tabulated on p. 143 can also be made, but they are not so likely to furnish the correct solution.

From what has been said in preceding sections of this paper, it is evident that there are not perhaps sufficient facts available to decide finally between the above two principal theories; the arguments for and against which are fully reviewed on p. 115 *et seq.* A previous remark might again be repeated here :—*everything waits upon a demonstration of the precise relations of fly prevalence with diarrhoea.* A theory such as the ground theory must necessarily rest for proof upon the exclusion of other more likely theories; and a demonstration that fly-carriers are responsible for a really considerable part of the epidemic cases would of course tend speedily to dissolve the claims and the necessity for the existence of the former hypothesis.

On the other hand, it is possible that both influences take some part in the matter; and from *the piled-up mass of argument in favour of case-to-case infection*, on p. 115 *et seq.*, it is impossible to avoid the conclusion that already the ground theory must be profoundly modified to accommodate these facts. But here a grave difficulty arises; for, the greater the amount of case-to-case infection admitted the greater difficulty is there in explaining the profound variations or limitations of prevalence produced by temperature; for a direct effect of temperature upon the infectivity of the organism during transmission (see *A* (iv) above) does not, at present, come within the bounds of known and proved facts; *and we are thus driven on, willingly or unwillingly, upon the fly-carrier theory*, which has already been shown capable of satisfactorily explaining the whole matter, and which is the only one appearing, at present, at all likely to do so. On the other hand, though the theory of case-to-case infection should be completely demonstrated, the precise method of transmission is a question altogether apart. Moreover, the evidence for fly-carriage is only of an inferential kind, and *we dare not therefore accept the fly theory without certain confirmatory evidence of a direct kind*, such, for example, as that to be obtained by the three crucial tests outlined on p. 108. Again, the possibility also still remains that ground influences may play a definite, if only a minor part, in producing a seasonal increase of infectivity in the organisms which the fly-carrier has the task of distributing.

(2) *The "Bacterial Content of Food" Theory.*

The bacterial content of food has been shown to vary directly with the degree of temperature (see p. 80). The fact, however, that the numbers of diarrhoea cases do not vary evenly at all times of the season with the temperature, does not do away with the possibility of the diarrhoea prevalence being largely determined by the bacterial content of food, where the causal organism is supposed to be a specific variety, not of general distribution. Thus, at the beginning of the season, a considerable *pre-epidemic period* might elapse during the multiplication and spread of the specific organism, before appreciable dissemination of infection was produced. Again, later in the season, the phenomenon of *epidemic exhaustion* might represent, in addition perhaps to some exhaustion of susceptible persons, exhaustion also of the function of infectivity, or of multiplication, of the specific organisms. As regards the evidence for case-to-case infection, it will be recalled that the major part of that evidence rested upon the grouping of cases in point of time and of place; and this is quite consistent both with a "bacterial content" theory and to some extent with a "ground" theory, where the causal agency is a specific organism not distributed in a widespread manner, but limited to certain small foci. Bacteria might gain access to the food by *dust* and *flies*, as well as by human agency—the theory admitting of a large amount of case-to-case infection. Variations of prevalence with temperature could be explained by acceleration or retardation of multiplication of the specific virus in food; as well as partly by effects upon fly prevalence. The moderate probabilities existing as to the correctness of this theory—and, to a less extent, of the ground theory—indicate the need, at present, of some reserve in drawing final conclusions as to the causation of diarrhoea.

(3) *Some other Theories.*

A few agencies might here be briefly referred to, such as *heat* and *fruit*, which may possibly exert influences, at least of a general kind, in the causation of diarrhoea, but which were dismissed in an earlier part of the paper (cf. VI, 3, p. 83 ; and p. 115) as factors not exerting any special influence of the kind. If heat has no direct disturbing influence upon the digestive organs in summer, it at least greatly stimulates fermentation or kindred processes in food, particularly in fruit and milk ; and the digestive disturbances due to the latter may have not improbably a good deal of influence upon diarrhoea prevalence, at least upon the total amount. It is also quite possible that such digestive disturbances may be the means of lighting up much old infection in chronic and recurrent cases at the beginning of the season.

The phenomenon of *symbiosis*, again, always contains interesting possibilities; and, although the specific organism of diarrhoea may not itself be derived from the ground, yet a symbiotic revivification of its infective virulence may be produced, within the body, by the entrance within the latter, at the beginning of the season, of certain saprophytic ground organisms which have themselves been exposed outside the body to and modified by the maturing temperature influences of the pre-epidemic period.

In conclusion, however, it is a question whether it will not be finally demonstrated that the influences determining the epidemic prevalence of diarrhoea are referable, not wholly to one, but to a number of, interacting factors. Thus, whether there is or is not maturation of a ground organism, there is not improbably in any case a certain amount of fly-carriage, of multiplication in food, and of direct personal infection ; as well as, possibly, some exhaustion of infectivity of the causal organism, beside the known and proved exhaustion of susceptible persons. It is important, again, to note that of the various theories as to method of spread, *the "fly-carrier" theory is, at present, the one best able to stand alone as a complete and all-sufficient explanation of the facts at present available.*

It may further be noted however that, as regards the importance of the part played by cumulative temperature effects or fly prevalence, *in starting* the epidemic, there is always the possibility that the influence of these factors may appear to be more important than it really is. The part they play may be one of minor importance; simply providing the match that lights up the conflagration in a great mass of susceptible material. The explosive violence of the diarrhoea epidemic, perhaps second only to that of measles amongst the commoner infectious diseases, should be here recalled, and particularly the violent up-rush in hot countries and the immediate falling away, as if the epidemic had over-reached itself, occurring months before midsummer is reached (cf. Chart B, p. 120, Melb.). Due importance must be therefore given to the great quantity of susceptible material that has been accumulating since the preceding epidemic, or to the possible alternative theory as to gradual recovery of infective virulence of the causal organism. It is not certain, however, that the rise in late seasons occurs in greater force on account of being greatly delayed. Conversely, the possibility might also be considered, whether, after a succession of seasons in which no epidemic has occurred owing to the complete absence of the necessary temperatures or again of fly prevalence, the diarrhoea prevalence might not force its way up in spite of the almost complete unfavourableness of the latter factors, owing to unwonted great accumulation of susceptible material or to the complete recovery of a high degree of virulence. It might thus be advisable to provisionally consider the influence of temperature or fly prevalence as to some extent a relative rather than as altogether an absolute deciding factor of the epidemic prevalence of diarrhoea.

VIII. Prevention and Treatment.

Were it possible to sum up the essential features of diarrhoea in a single sentence, without risk of misunderstanding, it might be said that epidemic diarrhoea is a disease of *young*, *healthy*, and *dirty* families. The apparent paradox which the second of these epithets presents has already been explained on p. 28: in the same sense as that in which the term is applied to certain acute specific diseases which notably affect a large number of healthy young persons, diarrhoea also is a "disease of health." The mortality alone is, however, largely confined to weak and ailing infants. From this latter fact the argument has been deduced that preventive measures tend only to retain within the population a large number of the "unfit," whose loss would rather be a gain than otherwise to the community. But it is only necessary to point, in answer to this, to the still large minority of cases which succumb to severe infective diarrhoea, who are physically of the soundest (cf. p. 29); and to the after effects in those who recover. That *diarrhoea calls urgently for measures to limit its yearly ravages* is evident from the three following important economical considerations:

(1) *It is the cause of a huge infantile mortality;* and moreover there is reason to think that the many deaths certified as due to " convulsions," " dentition," " marasmus," and other like ailments which, it is significant to recall, also show marked seasonal variations parallel with those of diarrhoea, are very often actual instances of diarrhoea, or at least are closely related to it.

(2) *The after-effects it leaves upon those infants who recover is probably an equally serious consideration.* Firstly, it should be noted that in the two areas an average of half the babies in each of the first three years of life were attacked during 1908, a year of only moderately high prevalence; so that it might be fairly assumed that almost all the babies born in these districts had diarrhoea at least once before reaching three years, and many of them on several occasions: a wholesale incidence which recalls the similar wholesale affection of the children of the coloured races with malaria. Secondly, serious impairment such as fibrosis of the organs of the body is said to follow and to make itself apparent in after life; which might indeed be expected from the serious lesions described by Ballard (1887–8, p. 15) in the cases examined. Thirdly, all this is well borne out by Newsholme (1909–10), who found that towns having high infantile mortality also had high mortalities at the later periods of life.

(3) *The great economic loss due to the illness and to its after-effects in adults,* who are frequently compelled to remain away from work for long periods (cf. p. 22); but not the least important, from the writer's observations, are *the immediate after-effects—the low state of vitality induced at the close of the autumn,* leaving both *adults* and *young children* an easy prey to the bronchitis and pneumonia of the cold weather which immediately follows.

Finally, to the above observations might be added that of the whole-sale incidence of this loathsome disease in certain parts of the country, *e.g.*, the yearly occurrence of about 3000 cases in a population of 33,000. Better warrant than such facts offer could hardly be desired for the in-stitution of wholesale preventive measures in a disease which is at once the scourge and the great sanitary reproach of so-called civilized lands.

1. *Treatment of Diarrhoea.*

As regards treatment, the various adjustments of the diet are useful, in great measure perhaps because they serve to pick out cases of irritative digestive disturbance, where the specific element is either little in evidence or completely wanting. And such procedures as infusion of fluids where there has been great watery discharge, and washing out of the bowel, are doubtless also of service. But where a severe typical attack has to be dealt with it is probable that, as in the case of specific diseases generally, it has to run its own course, and the hope of the treatment of the future must lie in some anti-specific procedure, such as preventive inoculation or administration of curative serums. Above all things the discovery of a powerful antitoxin would be gladly welcomed. The cloudy swelling and marked degenerative changes in the kidneys and other organs (Ballard, 1887–8, p. 13), along with the great depression, point to the production of a powerful toxin to whose agency the dangerous accompaniments of the disease are largely attributable. The sharpest and most serious attacks last only for comparatively few days, and several injections of an efficient antitoxin would serve to carry the patient triumphantly through. But not only would such an antitoxin be invaluable for saving life, it would also have an enormous economic value in alleviating the suffering and prostration of non-fatal cases. It was surprising to meet so large a number of adults, especially men, who had to stay at home from work on account of diarrhoea, the length of the detention being often a week or a fortnight. The prostration was also great, even to the point of danger to life; and in such cases one could not help thinking an efficient remedy, such as an antitoxin might provide, would have been a great boon.

Whatever advances in treatment may be reserved for the future, there is some reason to hope that a great deal can be accomplished in the way of prevention.

2. *Prevention of Diarrhoea.*

No attempt will be made to deal exhaustively with this question, but merely to comment upon a few matters which have come most into prominence during the course of the inquiries.

(a) *Notification of Diarrhoea Sickness.*

Apart from considerations as to the value of the opportunity given by notification for remedial measures, there is the practical question as to whether any really large part of the cases would thus be brought to light. This was another interesting matter kept in view throughout the inquiries of 1908. I found that medical advice was sought in 49 out of a total of 390 separate attacks in the two districts, or in 12%. The data on this point were not quite complete, but the proportion could not have been very much more: and that in districts where most of the people are in medical clubs, and are in the habit of seeking medical advice pretty freely! This is in itself confirmatory evidence of the indifferent light in which the gravity of the affection is viewed amongst the classes who suffer most from diarrhoea. Only this one-eighth of the cases applying for medical relief would thus, in the usual course of things, have been notified. But although only 8% of attacked persons over two years of age were found to apply to a doctor, yet in this, and perhaps most other towns, probably many times that number apply to a chemist, diarrhoea mixtures being in great request during the hot summer. Thus it is evident that any attempt to obtain full notifications of all cases might need to include notifications by chemists. On the other hand, the financial burden imposed upon local administrative bodies by notification of all cases, in towns where the latter might include 10% of the whole population, is practically prohibitive of the procedure; and, again, until this wholesale incidence is reduced to more moderate proportions it is doubtful if the money would not be much better spent upon measures directed against household dirtiness and, perhaps, fly nuisance. *Notification of infants only* might, notwithstanding, be completely practicable and eminently beneficial, as *under two years of age* they only include ⅓th of the total number of cases, and since it is amongst infants that the greatest susceptibility, as well as most of the mortality, is found. It is true that, with a view to eradicative measures, notification of older children and adults is desirable; for the passing on of infection from the parents to the young children must be borne in mind. Yet, on the other hand, recalling the great attraction for diarrhoea of houses containing infants, if the special incidence upon infants could be satisfactorily dealt with the strongest predisposing cause for spread of the disease would be removed.

As to the age limit of notification, it is obvious that, in the first place, cases under 12 months, amongst whom the high mortality occurs, should certainly be included. Children of from one to two years, however, also present special reasons why they should be included, since their susceptibility to attack is greatest of all, and they are apparently the chief means of carrying on infection from one season to another: a fact of the greatest importance, considering their very frequent association with infants under 12 months. The fact that at between two and three years also the susceptibility is very high, and still as high as in the first year, is a good reason for including children up to three years. *Where, however, the chief end in view is the lowering of infant mortality, or where it is necessary to proceed on economical lines, notification of those over one or two years* could quite satisfactorily be made *conditional upon there being an infant under one year present in the same household*: the protection from infection of those under 12 months being the main object to be kept in mind. As a practical point it is interesting to note that of all separate attacks in the two areas in those under two years of age, out of 74 instances, medical advice was sought in 27 $^0/_0$, as against only in 8 $^0/_0$ of those above two years of age.

The Notification of Births Act and the appointment of Health Visitors has furnished various ways and means of following the health of the infant from birth onward; but, notwithstanding, since the Health Visitors' calls are necessarily separated by intervals of at least some weeks or months, it is evident that some means of securing more prompt notification to the Health Authorities of the occurrence of diarrhoea amongst young children should be arranged.

Finally, although partial notification may be unsatisfactory as regards comprehensive preventive measures, yet the lessons imparted in the feeding, caring for, and protection of infants from infection, cannot fail to have a beneficial educative effect upon the mother, if not at the moment for the saving of the infant attacked, at least as regards preventive measures in the future.

(b) *Isolation.*

(1) *The precautions adopted with regard to the isolation of attacked persons* will depend to some extent upon the final verdict as to the relative importance of the parts played by direct personal infection and fly infection. It would be altogether premature to attempt to formulate final methods of procedure until then. Nevertheless, in the meantime, a number of precautions might be recommended provisionally, particularly as in any case they must follow along very similar lines. In the first

place, it would be wise in any case to separate the sick and the healthy as far as possible from one another. Due allowance must be made for the fact that the writer's conclusions upon this subject are not yet complete and mature, and may yet be subjected to very radical modifications; but in accordance with present conceptions of the disease, if asked to guarantee the preservation of an infant charge from infection, I should not for a moment think of allowing it to remain in the same house as a person attacked with epidemic diarrhoea, the risk of infective matter gaining access to it, whether directly or indirectly, being too great, even with the adoption of all ordinary precautions. Thus, when diarrhoea occurs in a household a susceptible infant should be sent away with its nurse. In the class of households above dealt with, where this would not be practicable, a large degree of isolation is still possible. Thus, the affected person and unaffected infant might be restricted to separate rooms, at the very least when motions are being passed. The Health Visitor might also advise special precautions with any young children affected in the early spring, who appear to be chronic or recurrent cases likely to provide centres of infection at the beginning of the diarrhoeal season.

(2) *Backyards-in-common* should also be discouraged in all house-planning schemes, even on general sanitary considerations alone. Such yards afford too great facility for intercourse between the members of neighbouring households, particularly between those of tender years. Not only diarrhoea, but other infantile disorders of non-school age, such as whooping cough and measles, undoubtedly owe their possibilities of spread largely to this means; and the writer has made some attempt to investigate this matter. As regards even diphtheria and scarlet fever, I have noticed that in such yards, in summer, the amount of close association of children is almost as great as it is while they are at school. The ideal of preventive work against infectious diseases of all kinds is to increase the distance between the various units of the population as much as possible, and this is best attained by securing in the first place the greatest degree of isolation of individual households from each other. In addition, there is the moral effect, with the greater privacy and independence enjoyed: all the households in one yard are apt to sink to the same level of carelessness.

(3) *The choice of a residence* is another matter of great practical importance; particularly as moving from house to house presents no difficulty to, and is almost an annual occurrence with, many people of this class. In cases therefore where the parents express some special

anxiety upon the matter, the practitioner should certainly advise a choice of residence where the mass influence, firstly of babies (cf. p. 51), and secondly of dirtiness (cf. p. 54), can be avoided. The eastern half of σ Street, with a complete absence of infants, and a high standard of cleanliness, illustrates the complete practicability of choosing such sites.

(c) *Cleanliness in the household.*

It has already been remarked how great a scourge a dirty household may become to the neighbours in the matter of diarrhoea infection. The comparison of "clean" and "dirty sections" (cf. Table XX *b* and p. 54) showed that, amongst the cleanest of houses not containing infants (indices 1 and 2), twice the proportion were attacked in "dirty" as in "clean sections." In other words, *seven of these houses, themselves models of cleanliness*, out of a total of 33 affected households, *would not have been attacked at all if their neighbours had been reasonably cleanly in their habits*; that is, after something has been allowed for the greater proportion of houses containing infants adjacent. The writer has felt it to be little less than a tragedy, in the following up of infantile mortality, to discover deaths from diarrhoea amongst poor but worthy people, where the cleanliness of the household and care in feeding are beyond all praise, but where the filth and accompanying disease of dirty neighbours has again and again rendered it impossible to rear a healthy offspring. Society has a right to protect itself, and in the near future will no doubt do so, against this danger from dirty people, even to the extent of compulsory legislation. The recent legislation leading to the organized visitation of homes by specially trained nurses, in connection with school medical work and also with reference to the care of infants, shows the willingness of the public to have their attention turned to such matters. It is interesting to note the present large administrative outlay upon cleanliness of children's heads, and to compare the relative benefits obtained from the latter with the great economical advantages which must result from radical treatment of household dirtiness—the rank soil so to speak in which alone diarrhoea can develop into the present wholesale scourge.

Allusion has already been made to the comparisons (pp. 63–4) which public health writers are in the habit of drawing between different towns as regards their diarrhoea mortality rates and the accompanying provision of w.c's or pail closets, and recently the central authorities have published matter of that kind with a view to drawing attention to the laxness of certain local authorities. Such comparisons usually include the factors of sanitary accommodation, and other generally recognized ones upon which official data are commonly available. Density of the infant population, and differences in case-mortality, have been noted above (p. 63) as two others to which attention should be called; also perhaps fly nuisance; and lastly, there is the important factor of household dirtiness. The addition of the latter perhaps makes the list of factors bearing on diarrhoea mortality almost complete, and it is interesting to speculate to what extent the establishment of local coefficients, or standards, for each of these factors could be systematically made, and thus a useful gauge of the local relations of infantile mortality and sanitary conditions be always at hand. A sanitary survey of towns throughout the country as regards household dirtiness, carried out if possible by the same observer, seems quite practicable, judging by the success and rapidity with which estimates were arrived at at Mansfield, and which were afterwards satisfactorily borne out by averages founded on the data of individual houses: and if the factor be as important as this inquiry appears to show, the establishment of a local coefficient, even if only made once for all, should serve many useful theoretical and practical purposes.

Inspectors are necessary whose duties should be largely those of supervision, directed to *the proper working* of the various sanitary fitments of the household. Perhaps a lacuna has hitherto been admitted here in the carrying out of inspectorial work. Having applied himself to the remedying of all kinds of structural defects and the institution of suitable drains and sanitary conveniences, the sanitary inspector has perhaps been inclined to leave these things thereafter to work themselves; but that they certainly will not do, in the slum portions of a town! It is not too much to say of localities with which the writer is acquainted, that the institution of water-closets in the dirtiest parts of the town is not a success! Full reasons for this have already been given in Sect. V, 3. Inspectorial supervision is therefore required; limited, if so desired, to the diarrhoea and typhoid seasons; and directed to securing proper working and due cleanliness of sanitary conveniences, particularly the removal of that film of faecal material which probably serves more than anything else to nullify the advantage of the water-closet over the pan closet.

A little gentle coercion might also be applied in regard to two other important matters: checking the careless disposal of the faeces of young children, above infant years: and enjoining the regular removal of food from the table between meals into a suitable pantry.

Inspectorial observations with regard to such matters can usually be made in these small houses without crossing the threshold of the dwelling; and, as a matter of practical detail, it will speedily become apparent that there are not a large number of houses which it will be necessary to trouble with systematic visits. Unnecessary intrusion of inspectors into the home is of course undesirable, but in this matter it is a question of the undoubted right of the public to protect themselves against the breeding of a deadly disease at their very doors.

It is not out of place here to refer briefly to the chance of securing general improvement in matters of household cleanliness, and the possibility of successfully inculcating such knowledge to the school child. A striking fact, which the writer regards as of the highest practical importance, is that dirty or clean housewifery almost invariably runs in families. That is to say, the clean housewife as a rule will be found to have had a clean mother; and her daughters in turn will almost certainly maintain similar cleanly habits. So very few exceptions were found to this rule, in numerous incidental enquiries, that it appeared probable that early training was powerful enough, more often than not, to overcome irregular atavistic tendencies to laxness in this respect. There is every reason therefore to expect the very best in present and future generations from the persuading of the school child into cleanly ways, and from the inculcating of the appropriate feelings of shame, or of emulation, in connection with such matters.

A convenient opportunity for instruction of the schoolgirl in matters of household cleanliness might be found in the projected lessons in mothering. The suggestion has been made that the public crèches offer very great facilities in this connection. Their establishment and extension into a kind of infant bureau is primarily an absolute necessity in the conservation of the infant life of large towns. But their usefulness may be greatly increased by adapting them as centres for the instruction of schoolgirls in mothering. It is unnecessary to enlarge upon the great interest young girls would naturally take in lessons of this kind; particularly if actually entrusted with the care of a baby, with its feeding, and with the cleanliness of its cot, clothes, and the part of the crèche in which it is located. No better opportunity for lessons in household cleanliness could be desired; and after all, the want of cleanliness in connection with babies, it seems, may prove to lie at the root of the question of diarrhoea prevalence.

Where, at the threshold of the home, the work of the supervising inspector might be advisedly relinquished, the work of the health nurse should be begun; and the chief of her duties for some time must be the education of the public, particularly of the young mothers.

(d) *Education of the Public.*

The popular apathy and ignorance with regard to this disease has already been discussed at length (cf. Sect. III, 1, p. 21). The chief points upon which instruction is required are the following:

(1) Instruction of the public as to the *specific* and *wide-spread* nature of the disease: its great economical disadvantages: the erroneous nature of popular theories as to fruit, teething, etc.; and the evil effects of the indifference resulting from connection of the disease with such trivial causes.

(2) The disease is *infectious*: a fact at present quite unappreciated.

(3) Infection is conveyed by the *stools*: risk of faecal pollution cannot be therefore too carefully shunned.

(4) The disposal of *faecal material in children* not old enough to use the w.c. requires the strictest attention—*especially in the diarrhoea season.*

(a) The child's chair should be placed in the w.c., or in some unused room apart from the general household, and the child trained to use it there.

(b) Amongst younger children, where the use of the napkin has been discontinued, the latter should be replaced during diarrhoea attacks, so as to reduce the possibility of accidental pollution of floors to a minimum.

(c) The napkins should be put in to soak in the w.c., or at least not in the scullery or living room, where contact may be established between them and food utensils.

(d) The napkins should always be completely covered with water, and the vessel itself covered over,—disinfectants might here be habitually used.

Similar precautions should be adopted in soaking in the soiled bedclothes, and in the cleaning up of polluted floors.

(5) Breast-feeding, and the proper care of food, are most important.

(6) Proper care of the external sanitary fitments of the household is essential.

N.B.—The above instructions are of course somewhat in advance of, and are not to be taken as, the approved conclusions of this paper. They, however, have doubtless as much warrant for their provisional adoption as, *e.g.*, the widely spread injunctions as to boiling of milk. And there is ample proof of the readiness with which, by a few years of persistent teaching, the public can be brought round to accept new standpoints of this kind, in the fact of the almost general adoption in this town of the latter procedure and of the modern feeding bottle. It is important to note how much the co-operation of the general practitioner has meant in such matters.

Some explanation is here necessary of the fact that it has been assumed throughout this paper that communicability is exclusively concerned with infection from the dejecta of attacked persons, without any direct proof having been given. The difficulty of imagining any other mode of infection in the circumstances, and the indirect support of all the facts of personal infection here detailed, appear to justify this assumption, at least in the present state of our knowledge. During the inquiry no effort was spared to trace out other possible modes of infection and unpromising clues such as concurrent sore throat were carefully followed up, bacteriological examinations being made in two of such cases (cf. p. 23).

(e) *Breast-feeding, and the Care of Food.*

Everything that tends to the cleanliness and sterility of food, including the boiling of food and protection from dust and flies, must present a bar to the ingress of infection. The boiling of milk is a question apart, owing to the implication of matters not clearly understood relating to destruction of vital properties and alterations in digestibility. Perfectly fresh milk is probably better left unboiled: there seem to be protective virtues in cow's or goat's milk taken directly after milking akin to those in human milk taken at the breast. The keeping of these animals therefore for the feeding of infants is, next to the engaging of a wet nurse, the most reliable preventive measure that can be taken; the former being generally the less expensive procedure. "Stale milk," on the other hand, that is, milk which has lost its first freshness, is perhaps better boiled, but it would be much better not to give it at all. Attention must again be called to the protective influence of milk taken at the breast—a fact doubly accentuated. Thus, up till 9 months of age it appeared that a breast-fed child could ingest almost unlimited quantities of household dirt with more or less impunity. Again, there is the curious fact in Table XIX *b* that breast-feeding saved more infants from attack in the dirtiest than in the cleanest houses. If then the necessity of having the milk newly-drawn is as great as it appears to be, measures directed to securing the immediate delivery of newly-drawn and unaltered milk would take precedence over all other processes aiming at purification or preservation; and the writer is tempted to suggest that of all the various systems of milk-supply with which he is acquainted, none more closely approaches this ideal than that which he has seen in one of the old suburbs of Paris—the goatherd leading his flock and milking them at the customers' doors. From the point of view of the infant, at least, nothing better could be desired, except that the first and last milks differ greatly in the percentage of cream. There is only one alternative to this—strict supervision and prompt delivery of milk, several times during the day, to houses containing infants under 12 months of age. To accomplish this successfully, public control of the milk-supply would probably be necessary. The wholesale prevalence in the quadrilateral district, notwithstanding the complete provision of water-closets and the habitual boiling of milk, is a sufficient commentary upon the fact that the institution of these procedures still leaves the principal causative factors of the disease practically untouched.

(*f*) *General Sanitary Measures.*

All the numerous sanitary measures dealing with the general planning of houses and their sanitary arrangements must certainly tend to lessen the incidence of diarrhoea. Thus, water-closets should undoubtedly give better results than pan closets or privies were they used in a careful and cleanly manner. There is a popular saying to the effect that dirty people can turn the best appointed house into a pig-sty; and it is evident from the results of this inquiry that this kind of social lapse is not without grave epidemiological significance.

The rapidity with which people in these mining and manufacturing towns of the midlands—where, incidentally, diarrhoea reaches its greatest prevalence—can turn fine blocks of newly built houses into what is virtually slum property, is little short of amazing. The conversion of the unused front sitting-room into a swimming pool for domestic birds has been noticed; as well as the refusal by a family, through laxity or ignorance, of the use of the water-closet, the pavements around the house being preferred. It has been thought necessary in several parts of the paper to detail a few of these persisting barbarisms, in order to avoid misunderstanding by those whose experience may be wholly confined to the cleaner rural counties of the south.

At the same time the writer would like to make it clear that Mansfield itself comes far from heading the list of the neighbouring midland towns as regards infantile mortality or household dirtiness. On the other hand, the midland mining towns are very much alike in these matters, a fact depending on the very similar characteristics of the collier population throughout. Of these towns it might be said that it is the people that live in the houses, and not the houses themselves, that are at fault, the latter being generally fairly new brick dwellings and built according to recent by-laws : being constructed again on a very similar plan throughout the mining districts.

The essential importance of the question of dirtiness is evident in the fact that it was found to apply in the whole field of sanitary provisions both within and without the house ; as regards the working of the w.c. (cf. p. 60); the yard-paving (cf. p. 57) and drains; in the care of food (cf. p. 56); and as regards faecal pollution within the house (cf. p. 56 *et seq.*).

All sanitary measures bearing upon the prevention of diarrhoea may therefore be arranged antithetically under the two following headings :—

(1) *General measures under public supervision* : with regard to proper house-planning, including suitable places for the storage and protection of food; satisfactory drains, w.c's, and ash receptacles; pure water, milk, and food supplies.

(2) *Particular measures within the home, at present left entirely to the caprice of the householders themselves* ; relating to the satisfactory working and application of the above general provisions, to the habits of living, and to the management of persons attacked.

While it would not be suggested that one iota should be abated of the many and various general sanitary measures that have over a course of several decades been put forward and applied in this disease, there is almost sufficient justification for declaring that *their beneficial influence may be completely neutralized*, and diarrhoea may rage with undiminished violence where there are

(*a*) Dirty and careless habits of living; including carelessness with food.

(*b*) Want of care in isolation of attacked persons and in the handling and exposure of their stools.

Again, the above facts might be profitably considered from another standpoint, the antithesis in this case being made between *public cleanliness* on the one hand, and *private cleanliness* on the other. Thus, by such general measures as the above the householder has been provided with clean air, clean water, milk, and food supplies, and with arrangements for the cleanly removal of all waste matters. But it is not sufficient to merely place these benefits at his door; it is necessary not to forget the important part assignable to private cleanliness; for dirty householders, if left to themselves, are able to rapidly and effectually undo all this public labour, grossly contaminating all pure supplies received into their homes.

To introduce the topic of "private cleanliness"—including cleanliness of the household and also of the person—is to open up a department of hygiene of immense extent. That it is also a still largely undeveloped field is suggested by the fact that one disease at least—epidemic diarrhoea—has been able, notwithstanding the adoption of numerous sanitary reforms, to securely maintain its footing, and also by the fact of the large number of previously unsuspected evils only now being revealed to the public by the institution of regular home visitation in connection with the prevention of infantile mortality and with the medical inspection of schools. It is important to note the long list of evils attendant upon dirty and careless habits of living. Thus, within the home there is the increased spread and higher mortality of most infectious diseases, particularly whooping cough, measles, diarrhoea, and other infantile complaints; the septic complications of scarlet fever, diphtheria, and of advanced phthisis are also referred to similar causes. Again, with regard to personal cleanliness, one fails even yet to fully comprehend or mentally fathom the depths of uncleanliness and neglect evidenced by the verminous state of the majority of the children in the slums of the large cities; and we may go even further and include matters of still more intimate personal concern, such as the question of oral sepsis from neglected teeth, with the vicious circle of throat troubles, impaired nutrition, and other evils following. Such recognition of the wideness of the bounds of this subject of "private cleanliness" is as a matter of fact of the greatest importance with regard to the prevention of diarrhoea; for it must be understood that all the various agencies, particularly through school channels, which are at present helping to raise the general standard of cleanliness throughout the community, are at the same time tending to bring the prevention of diarrhoea rapidly within the bounds of practicability. Without these indirect aids, the problem might have seemed quite hopeless. When we find however that with the comparatively recent institution of such agencies certain conditions of personal filth are already threatening to become rare, there is every reason to expect the best results from the education of the public in these and all kindred matters. Other points to be noted here are that the poor and dirty districts of a town have always constituted themselves, to a large extent, shelters or strongholds from which the various infectious diseases issue forth to ravage the community at large. Again, that notwithstanding ideal housing reforms, the dirty habits of the people may still persist. And that while the prevalence of certain diseases may depend primarily upon defective housing conditions, others, such as diarrhoea, may have their basis rather upon the habits of the householders themselves. The two districts were particularly interesting from the fact that the housing conditions were thoroughly good, and that the dirtiness one saw there was of the essential and inexcusable kind, altogether unqualified or unexcused by poverty or other depressing causes.

It is of course useful to be able to state the results of the inquiry in some such definite manner as the above, but it is only too evident on a perusal of the preceding sections that there are too many points connected with the causation of the disease yet in doubt to allow of anything final in the way of conclusions.

A demonstration as to fly-carriage would of course suggest measures against the multiplication of flies, by directing attention to the disposal of the refuse in which they breed. The points at which precautions against fly infection might be inserted in the foregoing considerations as to preventive measures are obvious enough to need no further remark here, except to note the necessity of securing that flies are not allowed to settle upon the lips of infants, or upon food, or infectious discharges. It is evident, however, that whether the fly theory be proved or not, the importance of the above summing-up as well as of other parts of the paper must still to a large extent hold good; *for flies can only become dangerous to any extent where there is laxity of the kind described in* (*a*) *and* (*b*). In any case eradicative procedures of the two kinds, as in malaria, should certainly go hand in hand.

Nevertheless, while the gradual inculcation and enforcement of cleanliness, and other measures, may lead to the levelling down of the greater part of the seasonal curve, yet the method of spread appears to be sufficiently independent of gross pollution to make it more than likely that a moderate incidence would still persist. Whether this does, or does not, depend upon the peculiar ability of a carrier, such as the fly, to deal with very minute traces of infective matter is not yet certain. It is possible that, with its constant journeyings to and fro and penetration into every part of the household, the fly might cause nearly as much disease by carriage from the almost microscopical traces of infection on the basin of an apparently clean w.c., situated within a clean dwelling, as from a pan closet also so situated. Wholesale reductions in the prevalence of flies might thus be essential to the levelling down of the last part of the epidemic wave: and *the levelling down of the epidemic wave to a straight line*, as occurs in cold seasons (cf. Chart B, p. 120, Newcastle 1907), *is of course the ideal of preventive measures to be kept in mind!* On the other hand, direct personal infection may prove to be responsible for a considerable liability to spread in an ordinarily cleanly household. The concluding paragraph of Sect. VII, 2 (*b*), should however be here recalled: to the effect that perhaps the bulk of infection classed under this heading would yield to scrupulous care in washing, and in the handling and disposal of infectious discharges.

It is not of course intended to convey in these remarks upon household dirtiness more than that the latter is but one of several important causative agencies of diarrhoea prevalence. There is a popular sentiment that every sanitary sin brings its accompanying punishment. In the case of bad water supply and drainage the correctional disease is cholera or typhoid fever; both speedily diminishing with attention to such matters. In the case of household dirtiness, and possibly also of carelessness with fly-breeding refuse, it is perhaps diarrhoea.

In concluding this paper, I must acknowledge my indebtedness to Dr Charles Wills for permission to publish the data, and for kindly interest taken in the inception of the inquiry: also to Mr Philip J. Shacklock for his valuable meteorological data. Notwithstanding the time already taken in the preparation of the paper, the statistical analyses have proved so exacting, and the scope covered by the inquiry is so great, that I can only regard it as a hasty and premature survey of the main facts; and must claim the privilege of considerably modifying if need be the conclusions arrived at at a later date; it is also obvious in many places that the data will admit of much further mathematical treatment. Now that the very numerous interacting and conflicting causative factors have all been finally passed in review, the constant tendency to the masking of the sharpness of contrast due to the effect

11—2

of any one of them acting alone will be best appreciated, as well as a final word of warning not to underrate the importance of the small margins therefore found in many of the tables. It might be noted that the conclusions from the 1908 data were matured and considerably increased in value by the opportunities for confirmatory observations in 1909. The paper might have been fortified had there been time by the inclusion of many actual instances, illustrating various important points, extracted from the original notes: these also, along with additional notes of other kinds, may possibly form the subject of a later paper. Further, in order to keep its length within reasonable bounds anything like an attempt to review current opinions or to provide complete references to the conclusions obtained by other writers has been rigidly avoided throughout. References are only made to those conclusions which mark certain definite evolutionary stages, on some of which it might yet be necessary to retreat.

The collection of the data was completed two years ago, and some of the conclusions as to personal infection and other matters were embodied in another paper (1908). Since November 1909 when a draft of the paper was first placed in the Editor's hands no material alterations have been made. In the meantime, a number of very valuable papers upon the same subject have appeared. Some of these have anticipated and also unwittingly traversed arguments, and in some cases illustrations, already included in this paper. As they are not included in the bibliography a list is given at the foot. They illustrate the trend of current opinion, and the first presents valuable morbidity data marking one of the recent notable departures in the literature, as also in our conceptions, of the disease, hitherto somewhat distorted by facts derived exclusively from the mortality data.

DAVIES. "Summer Diarrhoea and Notifications." A special report to Woolwich Borough Council. Jan., 1909.

VINCENT. "The Etiology of Zymotic Enteritis." A pamphlet. Feb., 1910.

SANDILANDS. "The Communication of Diarrhoea, etc." *Proc. Roy. Soc. Med.* Feb., 1910.

NAISH. "Summer Diarrhoea." *Public Health.* Feb., 1910.

HAMER. "Flies and Vermin." Report by the Medical Officer, London County Council. March, 1910.

NIVEN. "Summer Diarrhoea and Enteric Fever." *Proc. Roy. Soc. Med.* April, 1910.

IX. GENERAL SUMMARY OF CONCLUSIONS.

Only a general outline of the chief conclusions is given here: all important sections in the text have a summary attached.

(1) *Age Incidence: Prevalence and Fatality, etc.*

(*a*) *The age incidence* of the mortality and morbidity differ markedly; and it is interesting to note that so many differences exist in the disease, as studied from the latter two standpoints, that separate recognition like that accorded to two different affections is almost justified.

(*b*) *Prevalence and fatality*: in some midland towns the disease is a veritable scourge; 10 % of the population may be attacked during the season; the cases may number a hundred times the total of deaths.

(2) *Clinical Features, Immunity, etc.*

The clinical picture of the disease was not always complete, but association with other cases generally served to confirm the diagnosis.

The incubation period was often found to be from 6 to 30 hours in length; possibly it is sometimes longer.

The duration of attack and tendency to recurrence varied directly with the age, *i.e.*, with the susceptibility of the patient. There is probably a moderate amount of acquired immunity.

The mortality, which is almost confined to infants, is determined to a striking extent by previous ill health of the patient.

(3) *Social Relations.*

Occupation was not found to produce any effect upon the incidence of the disease, except by the possible influence of the close association of the men at their work.

School attendance probably has little effect on the spread of infection, owing to the small susceptibility of those of school age.

The sharing of yards-in-common apparently had a marked influence upon the spread, or limitation, of infection.

(4) *Sanitation.*

Dirtiness of the household increases the incidence of the disease, probably through carelessness in dealing with the excreta, particularly of young children (cf. Conclusions, pp. 53—57).

The provision of water-closets, good drains, refuse receptacles, and yard paving, is in all cases of no avail where dirty and careless habits exist.

The question of w.c. versus pan closet is, moreover, probably only of minor importance; faecal infection having most to do with pollution of the interior of the household by young children not old enough to use the w.c., or by involuntary passage of stools in children of more mature years.

(5) *Food.*

(a) *Human and Cow's milk in Infant feeding.* The comparatively low incidence upon the first year of life appeared to be due to breast feeding. With the substitution of cow's milk in the second year the maximum incidence is attained. Boiling the cow's milk gave no protection whatever.

(b) *The milk-supply* apparently plays no part, unless one of a general kind, in introducing diarrhoea into the home (cf. Conclusions, p. 82).

(c) *Infection within the home* is probably the commonest method of contracting the disease. Much infection is frequently contracted where milk is altogether excluded from the dietary (cf. Conclusions, p. 82).

(d) *Solid foods:* it is possible that, all other things being equal, no one kind of food is more likely to be a vehicle of infection than another.

(6) *Epidemiological Features.*

(a) *Personal Infection, Direct Personal Infection, Fly-Carriage, Ground Infection, etc.* It appeared not improbable that the phenomena of diarrhoea prevalence are almost wholly concerned with the local evolution of various infective foci, and a piled-up mass of evidence has been presented as to the bulk of infection being derived by transmission from person to person. Further, as regards the above four sources or methods of infection a great deal of evidence was obtained for, and none against, the first three; and practically none was found exclusively supporting the last (cf. Conclusions, p. 115 *et seq.*).

(b) *Factors governing Epidemic Rise and Decline.* In relation to both the temperature and fly curves, the diarrhoea curve shows: a delayed rise; variations corresponding with their variations; and a definite falling away from their declining curves. The explosive form of the curve suggests multiplication by case-to-case infection, with gradual exhaustion of epidemic potential. The correspondences of the diarrhoea and fly curves are such as to be quite compatible with the theory of fly infection. Direct evidence, derived from the performance of certain crucial tests, is however necessary before practical adoption of the latter theory is warranted (cf. Conclusions, p. 143 *et seq.*).

(7) *Prevention and Treatment.*

Treatment. Much might be expected from a remedy such as an effective antitoxin or antibacterial serum.

Prevention. There is good reason for believing that a great deal can be accomplished by the following preventive measures:

(*a*) *Notification of diarrhoea sickness*: notification, of a partial kind, is shown to be practicable, and useful.

(*b*) *Isolation of attacked persons*: generally practicable to some slight extent.

(*c*) *Cleanliness in the household*: particularly with regard to avoidance, or cleanly removal, of faecal diarrhoeal pollution.

(*d*) *Education of the Public* as to the specific nature, and infectiousness, of the disease; as to infection through stools, etc.

(*e*) *Breast feeding*, wherever possible; *and proper care of food*: failing the breast a wet nurse should be procured, or a cow or goat obtained; or again in default, only milk newly drawn, and given unboiled. No reliance to be placed on boiling stale milk, *i.e.*, milk which has lost its first freshness; *such milk is better not given at all.*

(*f*) *General sanitary measures* should be attended to; but however complete their provision, diarrhoea may rage with undiminished violence where their beneficial influence is neutralised by :—

(i) Dirty and careless habits of living; including carelessness with food.

(ii) Want of care in isolation of attacked persons, and in the handling and exposure of their stools.

It is not sufficient to merely establish good water-closets, drains, etc.: in dirty districts supervision as to their cleanly working is absolutely necessary.

A demonstration of fly-carriage would call for destruction of fly-breeding grounds, and for precautions against exposure of infective discharges, as well as of food.

TABLE XXVII b. Giving some original data for the individual houses of the two districts.

In the columns H = index numbers of Houses: the numbers of Attacked Houses being in italics.

,,   Dt = index figures of Dirtiness. Division into the 33 "Clean" and "Dirty" Sections of Table XX a are indicated in this column by small marks.

,,   F = the Number of Children per house: italics are used in Houses containing Infants (under 2).

The Triangular Area:

H	Dt	F	H	Dt	F	H	Dt	F	H	Dt	F	H	Dt	F	H	Dt	F	H	Dt	F
1	4	10	27	2	0	53	1	3	81	2	8	107	3	3	133	2	3	159	3	1
2	5	4	28	2	0	54	2	1	82	3	3	108	3	2	134	2	6	160	-	4
3	3	2	29	2	4	55	2	5	83	-	5	109	3	2	135	2?	4	161	2	5
4	4	2	30	3	6	56	4	5	84	4|3	3	110	3	8	136	3	5	162	2	1
5	5	7	31	3	0	57	-	7	85	3	2	111	3	3	137	5	7	163	2	2
6	4	1	32	3	4	58	4	9	86	3	0	112	3	3	138	5	1	164	2	4
7	4	5	33	5	5	59	3	2	87	3	4	113	3	4	139	5	4	165	3	2
8	5	4	34	4	3	60	3	1	88	2	2	114	2	2	140	1	1	166	3	1
9	4	4	35	3	1	61	3	1	89	2	4	115	5	8	141	1	1	167	2	1
10	2	6	36	3	6	62	3	10	90	5	5	116	3	6	142	3	6	168	-	9
11	3	2	37	2	1	63	3	6	91	3½	1	117	3	4	143	3	7	169	3	0
12	3	1	38	2	5	64	4	7	92	3½	8	118	2	3	144	3	2	170	-	1
13	3	2	39	2	7	65	-	6	93	3	9	119	2	3	145	3	3	171	2½?	1
14	3	3	40	2	3	66	3	7	94	3½	3	120	2	0	146	2	2	172	3	2
15	2	4	41	3	4	67	3	2	95	3½	6	121	2	3	147	2	2	173	2	2
16	3	1	42	3	1	68	3	6	96	3½?	1	122	1	2	148	2	4	174	2	2
17	1	1	43	3	1	69	3	1	97	3½	6	123	1	2	149	1½	3	175	3	3
18	2	4	44	2	4	70	5	6	98	5	6	124	-	0	150	1½	1	176	3	1
19	4	1	45	3	5	71	5	6	99	3½	7	125	4	2	151	1½	3	177	3	3
20	4	9	46	1	3	72	4	7	100	3½	4	126	4	3	152	3½?	1	178	1	1
21	2	2	47	2	4	73	4	4	101	5	1	127	4½	8	153	3½?	4	179	2	5
22	2	5	48	3	2	74	3	1	102	4	4	128	1½	1	154	3½	6	180	2	2
23	4	3	49	3	3	75	3	4	103	3½?	3	129	1	1	155	1	0	181	2	3
24	2	3	50	3	3	76	-	3	104	3½?	2	130	1½?	1	156	1	1	182	2	2
25	2	4	51	3	4	77	5	2	105	4	1	131	3	5	157	1½?	0	183	1	3
26	2	8	52	3	3	78	5	3	106	4	9	132	2?	2	158	1	0	184	1	3
						79	4	4												
						80	3	1												

The Quadrilateral Area:

No.			No.			No.			No.			No.			No.			No.		
4	4	2	34	2	1	64	4	2	94	3	1	124	2	1	154	1	6	185	3	1
5	4	4	35	1	0	65	3	4	95	4	8	125	—	2	155	3	3	186	2	2
6	3	5	36	2	1	66	2	1	96	4	7	126	—	1	156	2½?	2	187	2	0
7	3	2	37	2	2	67	3	4	97	5	6	127	1	1	157	1	6	188	3	0
8	2	1	38	2	3	68	2	1	98	3	7	128	2	0	158	3	3	189	—	3
9	2	3	39	2	2	69	1	0	99	1	2	129	2	1	159	2	1	190	3	3
10	2	0	40	2	2	70	5	1	100	4	3	130	3	2	160	2	4	191	—	1
11	4	2	41	—	5	71	4	1	101	2	7	131	3	6	161	3	1	192	1	3
12	3	2	42	1	1	72	3	1	102	—	3	132	2	1	162	4	6	193	1	1
13	2	2	43	2	5	73	2	3	103	1	3	133	2	3	163	2	1	194	1	4
14	—	4	44	2	1	74	3	4	104	2	2	134	2	3	164	—	2	195	1	2
15	3	1	45	2	0	75	—	1	105	2	2	135	2	0	165	2	0	196	2	2
16	4	5	46	1	3	76	—	2	106	2	2	136	2	2	166	2⅔	2	197	1	1
17	4	5	47	1	2	77	2	5	107	2	5	137	2	1	167	1	1	198	1	0
18	1	3	48	2	1	78	3	1	108	4	4	138	5	4	168	2	1	199	1	4
19	5	0	49	3	5	79	3	6	109	3	5	139	3	1	169	2	3	200	1	2
20	—	4	50	3	1	80	2	4	110	2	4	140	2	0	170	2	2	201	1	1
21	3	4	51	4	3	81	2	7	111	2	1	141	2	3	171	1	3	202	1	4
22	3	5	52	3	1	82	3	3	112	2	0	142	2	1	172	1	4	203	—	0
23	3	1	53	1	2	83	2	1	113	1	5	143	2	2	173	1	0	204	1	4
24	3	3	54	2	2	84	3	5	114	—	0	144	3	2	174	3	4	205	1	5
25	1	2	55	2	4	85	2	2	115	2	1	145	2	1	175	4	5	206	1	0
26	4	4	56	3	1	86	2	2	116	—	3	146	2	5	176	4	1	207	—	3
27	4	2	57	—	3	87	3	2	117	1	2	147	2⅔	6	177	2	3	208	1	5
28	4	4	58	1	6	88	6	2	118	2	3	148	2	0	178	2	2	209	1	8
29	1	2	59	3	2	89	2	3	119	3	0	149	2	2	179	1	4	210	1	6
30	1	3	60	2	4	90	4	7	120	7	1	150	1	1	180	—	0	211	3	7
31	2	3	61	3	8	91	1	1	121	1	3	151	2?	2	181	—	1	212	4	4
32	3	2	62	2	0	92	3	6	122	6	1	152	—	1	183	3	5	213	5	3
33	1	0	63	2	2	93	2	1	123	1	4	153	—	0	184	3	0			

With regard to the index figures for *Dirtiness*, the above list was only used for the construction of Tables XXVII and XXVIII in the text: the other Tables are founded upon the data collected towards the middle of the season, which excludes the doubtful ones to which a query is attached above, and also a few others.

Only a few houses contained 2 *children under 2 years of age*, viz.: In the Triangle, Nos. 1, 26, 84 and 110: In the Quadrilateral, No. 186.

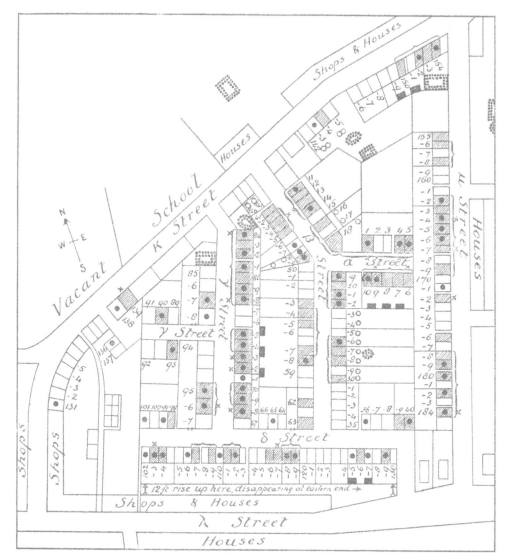

CHART I. *The "Triangular Area."* It has been necessary to simplify the Charts as much as possible: back entrances are only indicated in a few of the largest yards; in the others the entrance was generally tunnelled through the terrace from the front street: the projections of the rear premises (cf. Chart III), which were found practically throughout both districts, are levelled off here. Shops were not visited: houses not visited are not numbered: apart from this a few other irregularities have been admitted into the numbering. Areas I, II, and III are drawn to approximately the same scale.

Explanation of signs used.

▨ =	attacked houses.	▦ = privy-and-ashpit.
▢ =	unattacked houses.	⬡ = manure-heap.
▦ =	houses containing infants (under 2).	▩ = stable.
▢ =	when unnumbered = uncanvassed houses, or data are not complete.	⌢ = brackets enclosing "time and place groups" of Chart VII.
○○ =	pan (pail) closets.	×× = crosses are placed in the streets in front of houses in which cases had already occurred before July 3.

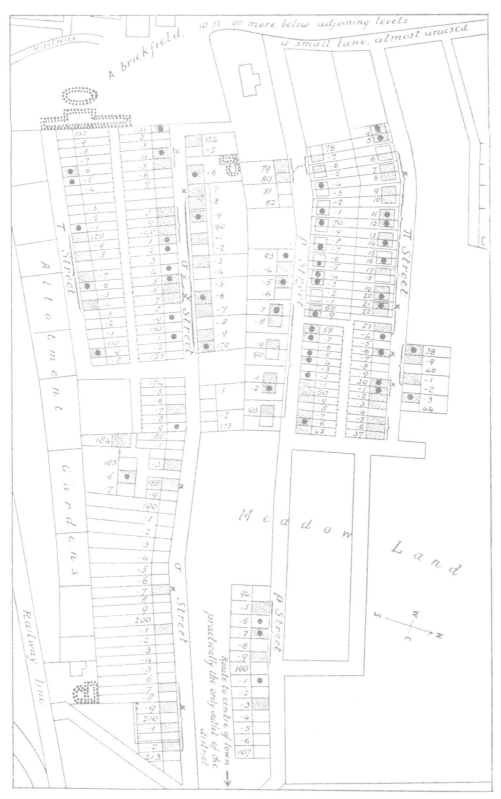

CHART II. *The "Quadrilateral Area."* (For explanatory notes see Chart I.) Open country bounds the district on the west and north, and a wide railway reserve on the south.

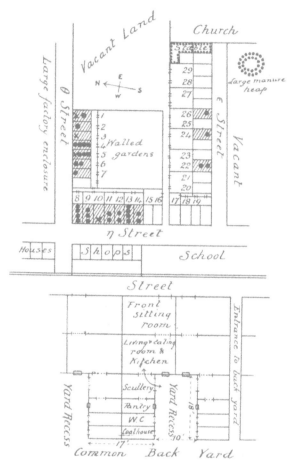

CHART III. (a) *"Area III."* Large fly-swarms were observed entering and spreading through the district from a large heap of horse-manure at the S.E. corner. Diarrhoea however appeared first in, and was almost confined to, the N.W. corner. No stables or breeding grounds for flies could be found anywhere around this corner within, at least, twice the distance separating it from the manure-heap at the S.E. corner. Other dwelling houses were also absent on all sides for considerable distances except immediately opposite the N.W. corner, from which direction then diarrhoea infection, if derived from outside, must have entered the district; *i.e.*, *against* the direction of the fly movements. Infection then, if carried between houses by flies, was not at least brought with them from their breeding ground. They were all new brick houses, with w.c.'s. Greater cleanliness and fewness of children did not explain the relative immunity of the houses in the S.E. corner. Cf. also Chart IV. The *signs used* are the same as in Chart I, except that ●=a diarrhoea case, × =a diarrhoea case occurring before July 18. (See p. 66.)

(b) *Plan of houses in a typical terrace.* Note the narrow recess at the rear, into which the kitchen, scullery, pantry, and w.c. of each pair of adjoining houses open. The measurements are merely typical. (See p. 35.)

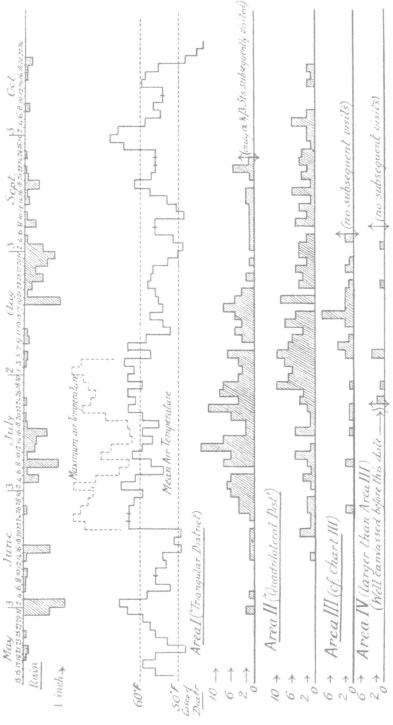

CHART IV. 2-day records of Onsets of Diarrhœa Attacks, and of Rainfall : 2-day averages of Mean and Maximum Air Temperatures : Mansfield, 1908.

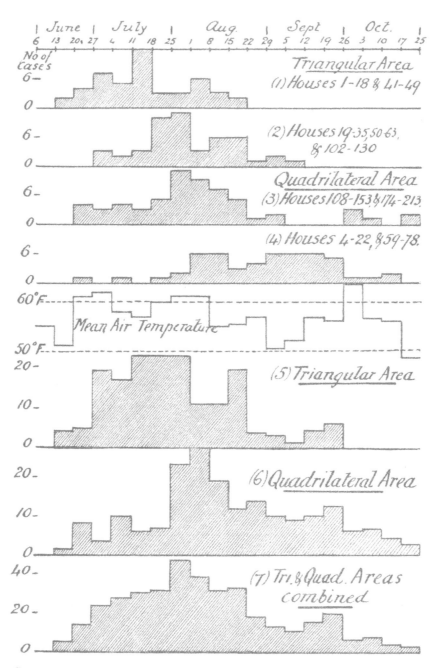

CHART V. *Weekly records* of Onsets of Diarrhoea Attacks, and of the Mean Air Temperature: 1908. Irregular evolution of the epidemic in different districts, epidemic exhaustion, and variations with temperature are well illustrated.

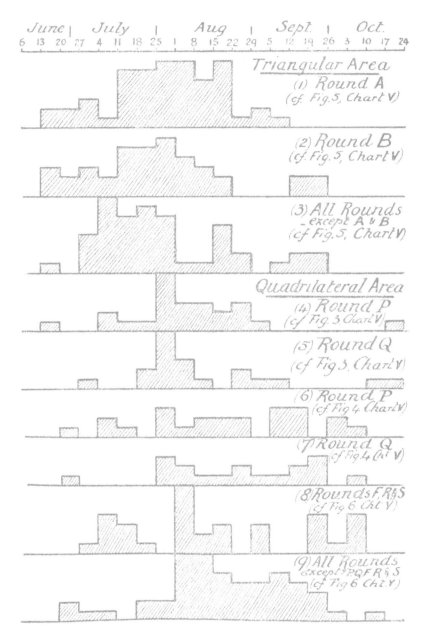

CHART VI. The number of attacks per week in various Milk-Rounds. Comparing the contour of the above figures with that of the corresponding figures in Chart V, and after making due allowances, remarkable correspondences in form are visible, the curve of attacks in any milk-round thus conforming with complete passivity to the curve of attacks in the whole section or district in which the milk-round is located; no part being therefore played by the Milk-Supply, unless one of a general kind, in the distribution of diarrhoea attacks. No suspicious clumping of cases was visible even when the daily records in each of the 21 rounds were separately examined. Rounds *P* and *Q*, to which special interest attaches, have been specially analysed. Figs. 6 and 7 include houses 4—78, and Figs. 4 and 5 the rest of the district. The drawing is to the same scale throughout: the maximum weeks of Fig. 1 are of 7 cases each. Cf. also Table XXXI, and p. 75 *et seq.*

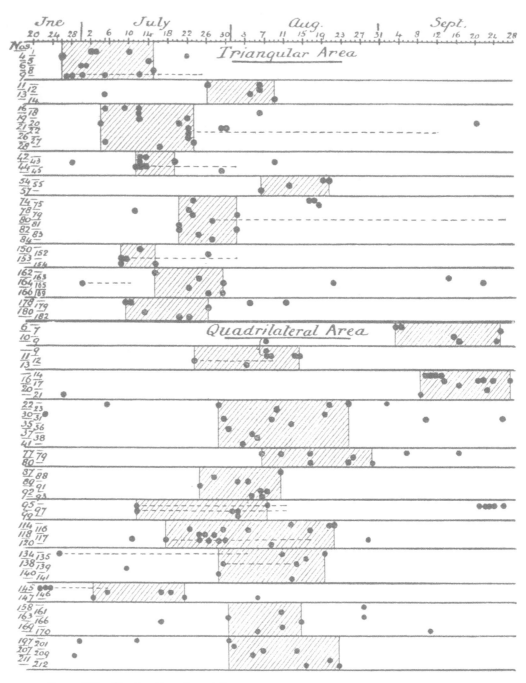

CHART VII. Showing Grouping of diarrhoea cases in point of Time, as well as of Place. The dots give the dates of onset of attacks when referred to the calendar at the top; the index numbers of the houses in which the attacks occur are also given in the left-hand margin: in a few cases, where of special interest, the length of the attacks is indicated by dotted lines. The above clumps are bracketed in Charts I and II. *All* attacks per house are indicated. With the exception of 58, triangle, and 76, quadrilateral, which should have been included above, there are 8 attacked houses in each district, included within the range of the attacked clumps, which are omitted for the sake of clearness: their attacks lie in every case outside the clumps, and as they average only about 2 attacks per house they did not, on a trial insertion, qualify in the least the very valuable demonstration of clumping in diarrhoea presented by this chart. Cf. p. 88.

REFERENCES.

ARMSTRONG, W. G. (1905). Some lessons from the statistics of infantile mortality in Sydney. *The Australasian Medical Gazette*, pp. 516—7.

BALLARD, E. (1887—8). Report on diarrhoea. *Supplement to the Annual Report of the Local Government Board.*

BOOBBYER, P. (1908). *Nottingham Annual Health Report*, p. 57.

BROWNLEE, J. (1905—6). Statistical studies in immunity, the theory of an epidemic. *Proc. Roy. Soc. Edin.* Vol. XXVI. Part VI.

BRUCE LOW (1887—8). An account of some instances of communicable diarrhoea, etc. Contained in the *Report on Diarrhoea* by Ballard (1887—8), p. 127.

DELÉPINE, S. (1903). The bearing of outbreaks of food poisoning upon the etiology of epidemic diarrhoea. *Journal of Hygiene*, Vol. III. pp. 68—91.

HAMER, W. H. (1908—10). *Reports on nuisance from flies, by the Medical Officer to the London County Council*, for the years 1907—8—9.

HOPE, E. W. (1904). *Liverpool Annual Health Report.*

JOHNSTON, W. (1878—9). The etiology of summer diarrhoea. *Trans. Epid. Soc.*, Vol. IV. Pt. II.

NEWSHOLME, A. (1902—4). *Brighton Annual Health Reports.*

—— (1906). Domestic infection in relation to epidemic diarrhoea. *Journal of Hygiene*, Vol VI. April.

—— (1909—10). *Thirty-ninth Annual Report of the Local Government Board.* Supplement to the Report of the Board's Medical Officer, containing Report of the Medical Officer on Infant and Child Mortality.

NEWSTEAD, R. (1907). *Preliminary report on the habits, life-cycle, and breeding-places of the common house-fly, etc.* Printed by the Health Committee, Liverpool.

NIVEN, J. (1904—6, 1908—9). *Manchester Annual Health Reports.*

PARK, W. H. (1901). The great bacterial contamination of the milk of cities. Can it be lessened by the action of health authorities? *Journal of Hygiene*, Vol. I. pp. 391—406.

PARSONS (1910). Discussion on summer diarrhoea and enteric fever. *Proc. Roy. Soc. Med.*, Epid. Section, June, p. 269.

PETERS, O. H. (1908). Season and Disease; a preliminary study. *Proc. Roy. Soc. Med.*, Epid. Section, November.

SANDILANDS, J. E. (1906). Epidemic diarrhoea and the bacterial content of food. *Journal of Hygiene*, Vol. VI. pp. 77—92.

STAWELL, R. R. (1899). Summer diarrhoea. *Intercolonial Medical Journal of Australasia*, March.

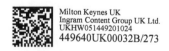